Epilepsy in Our Lives

Comments on *Epilepsy in Our Lives: Women Living with Epilepsy*

As a woman with epilepsy I will keep it with me for the support I need when next I encounter "the world that doesn't understand me."

A reader

I read *Epilepsy in Our Lives* and just wish books like this had been published when I was a kid growing up with epilepsy. It was wonderful to read about what others with epilepsy were experiencing that I could relate to.

A reader

Comments on *Epilepsy in Our Experience: Accounts of Health Care Professionals*

I felt very reassured knowing that other health care professionals have faced similar situations and am thankful for their willingness to share them.

A reader

This latest edition to the Brainstorms series undoubtedly will have many readers. All of them will be grateful to the editor and the fourscore contributors for the production of this unusual book.

Harry Meinardi, *Epilepsia*

Comments on *Epilepsy in Our View: Stories from Friends and Families of People Living with Epilepsy*

It sure would have been helpful for my wife and children to have read *Epilepsy in Our View* when they were first faced with the knowledge that their husband and father had a seizure disorder.

A reader

I would recommend that all patients with epilepsy own a copy of this book. It should also be included in medical bookstores and medical and community libraries.

Tonya F. Fuller, *Doody's Health Sciences Book Review Journal*

Comments on *Epilepsy in Our Words:*
Personal Accounts of Living with Seizures

You cannot imagine how much *Epilepsy in Our Words* has helped me to accept epilepsy as something I'm just going to have to live with. Just knowing that I'm not the only one that has gone through some of these experiences makes it easier.

A reader

. . . the first book of its kind.

USA Today

Comments on *Epilepsy in Our World:*
Stories of Living with Seizures from Around the World

This book is really wonderful! . . . Please receive all my congratulations for these books, for your continued project, your continuous learning and education how to understand, help, and treat people with epilepsy.

A reader

Comments on *Epilepsy on Our Terms:*
Stories by Children with Seizures and Their Parents

Thank you so much for your latest Brainstorms book. I have just finished reading it and I must tell you that I felt every emotion imaginable. Some of those children seemed to have a better grasp of their situation than I have. I cried, I laughed, and experienced all the feelings in between. The parents' stories were truly heartbreaking. To watch your child go through everything that epilepsy brings with it must be a horrifying thing. Most told their stories in such a realistic way that I had a mental image of just what they were going through.

A reader

To my knowledge, this is the first time families express themselves in detail and can express how the disorder is perceived "from the inside." Such an approach should prove most useful for the newly affected families who are suddenly faced with a disorder they had never heard of and who discover that their child has this mysterious disease.

Olivier Dulac, *Epilepsia*

Other Brainstorms books

Epilepsy in Our Experience:
Accounts of Health Care Professionals

Epilepsy in Our View:
Stories from Friends and Families of People Living with Epilepsy

Epilepsy in Our Words:
Personal Accounts of Living with Seizures

Epilepsy in Our World:
Stories of Living with Seizures from Around the World

Epilepsy on Our Terms:
Stories by Children with Seizures and Their Parents

Epilepsy in Our Lives
Women Living with Epilepsy

Steven C. Schachter, MD

Director of Research
Department of Neurology
Beth Israel Deaconess Medical Center

and

Professor of Neurology
Harvard Medical School
Boston, Massachusetts

Kaarkuzhali Babu Krishnamurthy, MD

Director, Women's Health in Epilepsy Program,
Comprehensive Epilepsy Center
Beth Israel Deaconess Medical Center

and

Assistant Professor of Neurology
Harvard Medical School
Boston, Massachusetts

Deborah T. Combs Cantrell, MD

Director and President of the Seizure, Neurological Disorders Center and
Director of The North Texas Epilepsy and Pregnancy Clinic,
North Texas Neuroscience Center
Irving, Texas

With Forewords by
Jackie Nink Pflug and
Kaarkuzhali Babu Krishnamurthy

OXFORD
UNIVERSITY PRESS

2008

OXFORD
UNIVERSITY PRESS

Oxford University Press, Inc., publishes works that further
Oxford University's objective of excellence
in research, scholarship, and education.

Oxford   New York
Auckland   Cape Town   Dar es Salaam   Hong Kong   Karachi
Kuala Lumpur   Madrid   Melbourne   Mexico City   Nairobi
New Delhi   Shanghai   Taipei   Toronto

With offices in
Argentina   Austria   Brazil   Chile   Czech Republic   France   Greece
Guatemala   Hungary   Italy   Japan   Poland   Portugal   Singapore
South Korea   Switzerland   Thailand   Turkey   Ukraine   Vietnam

Copyright © 2008 by Steven C. Schachter

Published by Oxford University Press, Inc.
198 Madison Avenue, New York, New York 10016
www.oup.com

Oxford is a registered trademark of Oxford University Press

Library of Congress Cataloging-in-Publication Data
Epilepsy in our lives : women living with epilepsy /
edited by Steven C. Schachter, Kaarkuzhali Babu Krishnamurthy,
Deborah T. Combs Cantrell.
p. cm. — (Brainstorms ; [5])
Rev. ed. of: The brainstorms woman / edited by Steven C.
Schachter, Lisa F. Andermann. c2000.
ISBN 978-0-19-533086-1
1. Epileptics—Biography.   2. Women—Biography.   3. Women—Diseases.
[DNLM: 1. Epilepsy—Personal Narratives.   2. Women—Personal Narratives.
WL 385 E64125 2007]   I. Schachter, Steven C.   II. Krishnamurthy,
Kaarkuzhali Babu.   III. Combs Cantrell, Deborah T.   IV. Brainstorms woman.   V. Brainstorms series ; 5.
RC372.3.S33   2007   362.196'85300922—dc22   2007016926

Cover Art: Leonard Lehrer, an artist whose daughter, Anna-Katrina, had epilepsy
http://work.colum.edu/~llehrer
Maestá, mixed media on panel, 48 × 36 inches, 1996
Maestá (Italian for Majesty) is the title of early Renaissance painter Duccio's remarkable masterwork in Siena:
a multi-paneled, partially medieval and partially Renaissance, series of images celebrating biblical sagas.
Anna-Katrina, daughter of Marilyn and Leonard Lehrer, was a child of many special needs. In the face of great
barriers she lived a beautiful and productive life and produced a group of poems, many paintings and
served as an inspiration to many. *Maestá* is intended to be a visual celebration of Anna-Katrina's remarkable life.
Artist Leonard Lehrer, who has exhibited internationally, is represented in many major museums and
collections in the US and abroad, and has been awarded numerous prizes including two
Fulbright Senior Scholar Awards to Greece. He lives and works in Chicago.

1 3 5 7 9 8 6 4 2
Printed in the United States of America
on acid-free paper

To all women with epilepsy—past, present, and future

Contents

Foreword by Jackie Nink Pflug   xi

Foreword by Kaarkuzhali Babu Krishnamurthy   xv

Preface by Steven C. Schachter   xxi

Contributing Authors   xxv

Personal Stories   1

Glossary   123

Index   127

Foreword

I was touched by the request to write a foreword for this book and am truly honored to share the same pages graced by the words of so many wonderful contributors.

Very few phrases change your life like "You have epilepsy." But now, more than 20 years after receiving my own diagnosis, I can honestly tell you that the condition has led me down a wonderful path. Along the way, I have encountered some of the most incredible people that I could ever hope to meet. One of these people is Dr. Steven Schachter, the driving force behind the *Brainstorms* series. Another is my neurologist, Dr. Ilo Leppik, from the Minnesota Comprehensive Epilepsy Center, who remains a loyal and steadfast contributor to both my seizure control and my emotional stability.

For me, epilepsy wasn't the end, but in many ways part of a new beginning. You see, put in context, my diagnosis of epilepsy wasn't a single, life-altering event, but a link in a chain of cascading events that resulted from a horrific tragedy that I suffered nearly 21 years ago.

In 1985, I was 30 years old and one of three U.S. citizens aboard an Egyptian airliner bound for Cairo. Shortly into its flight, the plane was forced to land abruptly by gun-and-bomb-wielding terrorist hijackers. Because authorities did not meet the terrorists' demands, they began to execute the passengers on board, one by one. I was the fifth person to be shot in the head at point-blank range. I was then shoved out of the plane onto the tarmac and left for dead.

But rather than die on that tarmac, I lived. The brain trauma that I suffered from the bullet caused epilepsy. After learning the diagnosis, I investigated every option for treatment, trying to find a therapy that felt right for me. That's when I met Dr. Leppik and reached my goal.

Since then, I wrote about my experiences in a book entitled *Miles to Go Before I Sleep: My Grateful Journey Back from the Hijacking of Egypt Air Flight 648*. I also met and married a wonderful man named Jim, gave birth to a healthy baby boy, Tanner, and launched a career as a motivational speaker in the hope that others can learn from my experiences.

No, I am not "cured" of my epilepsy, nor am I cured of my fears. While I have healed physically, I know in my heart that my healing is a process that is never fully completed. I am not the same person I was before the hijacking. And I am honestly *grateful* for that, because I have learned so much. I will never let myself stop learning and growing.

Dear readers, as you face your own uncertainties with epilepsy, try to remember what I now know: Everything happens for a reason, and something good always comes out of what appears to be bad. Remember that you have what it takes deep inside to cope with your condition and overcome your fears.

The road may be filled with unexpected turns. But no matter where your journey leads you, don't ever forget to take care of yourself. Be good to yourself. Be true to yourself. And most of all, remember to love yourself.

Jackie Nink Pflug

Foreword

Women with epilepsy have unique concerns about their lives, some of which begin at the moment of diagnosis. When should I tell a prospective boyfriend or partner that I have epilepsy? Will they be scared off? Will my children be born with birth defects? Will they have seizures? Will I be able to get and keep the job I want?

Historically, women with epilepsy have faced discrimination—at home, in the workplace, and in the doctor's office—that often influenced their living conditions and the evaluation and treatment of their medical condition. Before the nineteenth century, the cause of epilepsy in women was believed to be demonic possession. Later, the correct observation was made that some women had seizures related to the timing of their menstrual cycle. However, this led to the conclusion that abstinence from sexual activity or removal of the uterus or ovaries would cure epilepsy!

Fortunately, our current understanding of the relationship between epilepsy and the hormones that control the reproductive system is much further advanced and continues to grow. We know that many women with epilepsy have their first seizure around the time of menarche, when hormonal cycling begins and the first menstrual period occurs. We know that the balance between estrogen and progesterone, the two main hormones that control menstrual cycles, can influence seizures. Estrogen tends to provoke seizures in women who are sensitive to its influence, while progesterone can be protective. There are two times during a regular menstrual cycle when there is relatively more estrogen than progesterone—at the time of ovulation and around the time of menstruation. Some women experience most of their seizures around these two times of their menstrual cycles.

Other women may have menstrual cycles during which ovulation does not occur. That is, an egg is not released by one of the ovaries as normally happens mid-cycle. This can make women prone to seizures during the entire second half of the menstrual cycle. They may also have difficulty becoming pregnant, because conception requires ovulation.

Women with epilepsy are often reluctant to discuss their sexuality and the related issues. They may be afraid of having seizures in the setting of intimacy. They worry about telling prospective life partners that they have seizures for fear that this may drive them away. Because of these fears, some women with epilepsy may avoid marriage or pregnancy. Simply being advised by a health care provider or team of professionals that fears like these are common and generally unfounded may help women overcome their concerns and enjoy more fulfilling intimate relationships.

Birth control is another important area of concern. Oral contraceptives may increase the chances of having seizures, particularly those with high concentrations of estrogen. In addition, some of the seizure medications cause the liver to metabolize (break down) hormonal contraceptives at a faster rate than usual, leaving women less protected from becoming pregnant. Many women with epilepsy, however, are not adequately informed about these risks. They should be told that the use of barrier methods, such as a diaphragm and condom, can add to the effectiveness of standard hormonal contraceptive methods.

Pregnancy can be a wonderful time for women, but a frightening prospect for those with epilepsy. Some caregivers incorrectly tell women with seizures that they should never get pregnant, because seizure medications have a high likelihood of causing birth defects in babies.

The fact is that women with epilepsy have more than a 90% chance of having a normal, healthy baby. The chances for giving birth to a baby without birth defects are enhanced by taking the fewest number of antiseizure medications necessary and at the lowest doses required to maintain good seizure control, even before conception occurs. Daily folic acid supplementation can be of additional value, possibly because some seizure medications may interfere with how the body uses folic acid. Studies in healthy women have shown that folic acid supplementation for the first 6 to 8 weeks of fetal life can reduce the chances of particular birth defects that affect the brain and spinal cord.

As a woman goes through pregnancy, her metabolism and body weight increase. Both of these changes result in the need for higher daily dosages of seizure medication(s). It is essential for the pregnant woman, her obstetrician, and her neurologist to all work together to try to adjust doses of medication in conjunction with these changes, so that breakthrough seizures are less likely to occur. Also, this team approach can help to prevent seizures from occurring during labor and delivery.

After delivery, fluid shifts and hormonal fluctuations, in addition to the fatigue from childbirth and subsequent sleep deprivation, can increase the risk of seizures. Careful monitoring of blood levels and lifestyle modifications can reduce this risk significantly.

For most women with epilepsy, breast-feeding is possible and poses no significant risk to their babies. Some women choose a combination of breast and bottle feeding, thus allowing family members to feed the baby at night. This gives the mother more sleep, lessening the risk of seizures from sleep deprivation.

A woman's seizure pattern may change with the approach of menopause. Before the levels of estrogen and progesterone ultimately decrease as menopause ends, they may fluctuate rapidly for up to 2 years, causing more difficulty with seizure control. For some women, careful replacement of these hormones can restore good seizure control. For others, adjustment of the doses of seizure medications may help. This is another time in a woman's life when good communication between the patient, her internist or gynecologist, and her neurologist is necessary.

Another problem for women with epilepsy is the potential long-term effects of seizure medications on bone density. Some of these medications appear to increase a woman's chances of developing osteoporosis, or brittle bone disease. The key is to start taking preventive measures early—when seizure medications are first prescribed. A diet high in calcium, regular physical exercise, and avoidance of smoking and alcohol use are important because they may help prevent osteoporosis.

These are some of the many issues that are raised in this book. Effective communication is absolutely essential to address these issues. Women with epilepsy need and deserve to have as much information as possible regarding the effects of seizures and medications on their epilepsy, their pregnancies, and their bodies. They should feel comfortable discussing any or all of these concerns with their doctors, nurses, and other health care professionals.

At the Beth Israel Deaconess Medical Center in Boston, this communication is fostered by the Women's Health in Epilepsy program, founded in 1996. This program brings together members of the Comprehensive Epilepsy Center—epileptologists, epilepsy nurse specialists, neuroendocrinologists (experts in reproductive hormonal function), neuropsychologists (specialists in cognitive functions, such as memory), psychiatrists, social workers, and resource specialists—with general internists, obstetrician-gynecologists, a bone density expert, and an ethicist. Patients who enter the program are given access to members of the treatment team based on their individual needs. After each visit, progress notes are sent to each specialist, as well as to the patient herself, so that she remains an active partner in her health care.

As both our program and this book demonstrate, enabling women with epilepsy to share their experiences encourages others in similar positions to seek out information and work toward solving their problems. Without these connections, women may feel powerless and that they have no control over their lives. Information is power; with power comes control. The information in this book helps to make it possible for women with epilepsy to become more involved in their health care and to take control of their lives.

Kaarkuzhali Babu Krishnamurthy

Preface

Epilepsy in Our Lives: Women Living with Seizures. The fifth in a series of books about the individual and interpersonal aspects of seizures and epilepsy, focuses on women with epilepsy.

The medical profession has begun to appreciate the unique concerns of women with epilepsy and the connections between their seizures and reproductive hormonal function. Women, of course, have long understood these issues and physiologic connections; however, their personal perspectives have received relatively little attention in the medical and lay literature. It seemed to me, therefore, that their stories would add an important perspective to the Brainstorms series. The result is this volume.

I invited two colleagues who are known particularly for their work in this field, Drs. Kaarkuzhali Babu Krishnamurthy and Deborah T. Combs Cantrell, to assist me in asking women to write about their life experiences with epilepsy. The number of stories that we received was overwhelming, and the writings confirmed our impressions that women with epilepsy had a great deal to say to each other, their families, and the medical profession.

These heartfelt narratives embrace a wide range of topics. The impact of seizures on normal social development and growth, interpersonal relationships, reproductive hormonal function, and self-esteem is discussed in detail. Concerns about pregnancy, motherhood, loss of independence, and whether to disclose the diagnosis of epilepsy to significant others, friends, and employers are also covered. Finally, many of the writers express their frustrations about finding caring physicians who are knowledgeable about the unique issues faced by women with epilepsy.

As in the other Brainstorms books, the contributors have unselfishly bared their souls by writing with frank openness about their successes and failures, and joys and pain. I am deeply grateful and admire each of them for their determination and self-dignity, which propel them beyond the enormous obstacles placed before them by their disorder.

The primary purpose of this book is to present the perspectives of women of all ages who have epilepsy. It is intended for other women with epilepsy, their families and friends, and health care professionals. I hope that the insights of the contributors inform, encourage, and motivate readers. I hope as well that these stories open and strengthen communication between patients and health care providers and between women with epilepsy and their friends and loved ones.

This book includes two forewords. The first is a personal story by Jackie Nink Pflug about her recovery from an attempted execution during an airline hijacking and her subsequent triumph over epilepsy. Her resolve and spirit were tested by ordeals that few others will ever endure, and her courageous efforts to communicate her experiences have inspired countless others to overcome barriers in their lives. The second is an overview of the interconnections between seizures and reproductive hormonal function by my colleague Dr. Krishnamurthy. At the end of the book is an appendix prepared by Dr. Combs Cantrell that provides a glossary of many medical terms found throughout this book.

Many thanks to Cecile Davis for typing each of the stories, advising me, and keeping me organized and focused. Finally, I must thank my wife, Susan, who long ago taught me the value and importance of listening to women.

I invite those readers who would like to share their own stories or their reactions to this book to write to me at Beth Israel Deaconess Medical Center, East Campus, 330 Brookline Avenue, K-478, Boston, Massachusetts 02215.

Steven C. Schachter
March 31, 2007
(my wife's birthday)

Contributing Authors

Steven C. Schachter, MD
Director of Research, Department of Neurology, Beth Israel Deaconess Medical Center; Professor of Neurology, Harvard Medical School, Boston, Massachusetts

Kaarkuzhali Babu Krishnamurthy, MD
Director, Women's Health in Epilepsy Program, Comprehensive Epilepsy Center, Beth Israel Deaconess Medical Center; Assistant Professor of Neurology, Harvard Medical School, Boston, Massachusetts

Deborah T. Combs Cantrell, MD
Director and President of the Seizure, Neurological Disorders Center and Director of The North Texas Neuroscience Center, Irving, Texas

Personal Stories

1

(Age 26) Ever since I found out that I have epilepsy, I was told that having children might be dangerous for me. I met a nice person and ended up marrying him, but after what I had been told all my life, I was afraid that I wouldn't be able to give him what he desired so much: kids.

The idea of pregnancy scared me quite a bit. I kept telling myself "What if the child has birth defects? I will always blame myself." And this fear was is in addition to the thought that I might not be able to get pregnant at all. I had very irregular menstrual cycles, so I wondered whether pregnancy was physically possible for me.

And so, after dwelling on my limitations as a woman for so long and concluding that I was not "good" for my spouse, I initiated a divorce. Somewhere deep inside I understood that I first had to be comfortable with who I was, limitations and all. Only then could I ask someone else for understanding.

You see, I was always afraid of admitting that I had epilepsy to other people. My seizures usually went unnoticed by other people. That's why it was easier for me not to be open about my epilepsy, hoping that everyone would think that I was "normal." My ex-husband only found out that I had seizures almost 2 years after we started to date (we were not married yet). I am shocked now to realize how long it took me to actually tell him.

My first marriage showed me that you couldn't hide such an important part of yourself. That's why I told the first person that I seriously dated after my divorce about my epilepsy after 1 month. If someone couldn't handle that, I'd rather know about it sooner than later.

I can't talk to everyone about my seizures, but it was a huge step for me to actually "come out from my closet" and admit that I have this disorder. What I know now is that this experience is a part of healing. What helped me was attending a support group for women with epilepsy. I am very grateful for that. In the beginning, I was reluctant to share my experiences and fears, but I've learned that sharing is the whole point. And to think that I always thought it was crazy to do things like that. I've found out that I need support... as much as I can get!

I am still too sensitive at times. I find it difficult to live with epilepsy because I don't want to put the burden on anyone else's shoulders, like having to rely on other people to drive me places. This has been a problem when it comes to finding work. I am lucky that people don't judge me or label me just by my appearance, so job interviews are not a problem. But what is difficult for me is the location of the company or institution. I have had to say "no" to some very good job offers because of my inability to get there by public transportation.

If you ask me today what my dream is, I will tell you "to be free!" Do I understand the meaning of these three words? Am I not free now? I am learning how to enjoy myself, how to live in the world knowing my limitations. Yes, epilepsy is a part of me. I am stronger because of it, I am kinder because of it, and I am more understanding and less judgmental because of it.

2

(Age 53) Seizures and dating were never issues for me before I met my first husband. Up until then, I had male friends but few romantic attachments. I was too busy doing other things. Additionally, I hadn't met anybody on whom I was truly willing to spend time and affection.

In high school, I had a small circle of best friends—girls—who, like me, found the boys around us boring. However, we did find classical music concerts, art exhibits, lecture series, and planning our future careers exciting. Each of those friends eventually married—and remain married to the person they fell in love with at first sight.

I have kept in touch with these friends since our graduation from high school 35 years ago. They all have stories about me that begin: "Do you remember when you...?" No—I don't remember, but I don't mind that they remember. How could they forget? The stories they recall are striking and have weirdly funny aspects. My friends and I all have Central or Eastern European backgrounds, which may account for the part humor plays in our views of the world and for the *schadenfreude* that marks our humor.

But how could *I* forget? The stories all concerned my episodes of complex partial seizures, and I had no recollection of any of them. Until we were adults, none of my friends knew that I had epilepsy. They simply attributed my occasional bizarre behaviors to a combination of high intelligence and artistic gifts.

In fact, it took years before I was diagnosed with epilepsy. It was only after being shipped to the emergency room after suffering a grand mal that I was put on medication. This did help to control my grand mal seizures, but didn't do much else. My first husband always said that if I'd been male, I would have obtained good medical care right away. However, three decades ago, the old prejudice apparently still prevailed: men have medical problems; with women, it's all in their heads.

I believe I've led a charmed life. In school, at university, and later, I've always been able to make and keep good friends who accept me as I am. I do realize that being a friend to someone and living in the same house with them are two very different things, but my family was also a great source of strength in that regard. No one at home held me responsible for my seizures, but they held me

Personal Stories

accountable indeed for my nonseizure-related behavior. They also taught me, for example, to concentrate on my abilities rather than to see myself primarily in terms of my disability.

My first husband was a brilliant, gifted, insightful man with a superb sense of humor and a heart filled with kindness. I've never before or since known anyone with so little emotional baggage. He ran his own business from the house; I worked—also from the house—as a textile artist. He often found my seizure-induced behavior and my sudden, sharp mood swings to be difficult and painful. He remarked once, though, that while the bad times were bad, the good times more than made up for them. We had a wonderful life together for 14 years until his early death.

After my first husband died, I used what insurance money there was to pay tuition to finish up my fine arts studio training. Money from the sale of the business provided living expenses while I attended college full time. After that, I had to support myself.

I knew that to go on with my life, I had to take another medication that would control my seizures better. This meant a referral to a neurologist. I gave the internist treating me a list of specifications: the neurologist you refer me to has to be thus and so. (The only stipulation I recall now is "cannot be over thirty years of age.") The internist came through with flags flying to the accompaniment of a trumpet fanfare.

I was able to work and support myself. Because my seizures were almost invariably an evening-into-nighttime phenomenon and because I usually worked the day shift, I didn't experience many epilepsy-related job problems. I made career changes because of the changing economy more than anything else.

Two years after my first husband died, I met a very nice man on the commuter train. We agreed to meet daily on the train. One night, we were to attend a function together. We never made it. I suffered a complex partial seizure right in front of that nice man.

After I recovered, I thought for sure this would be "goodbye." It wasn't. We've been married now for 13 years.

Several years after our marriage, we went to see an obstetrician to talk about having a child. He considered out loud and in front of us the issue of a severely epileptic woman becoming pregnant and proceeded to plunge into a maelstrom of worry and doubt. My husband and I did not allow ourselves to be sucked in because we were determined to go forward and have a child.

My neurologist was our firm mainstay. Our attitude was that even if the developing baby showed signs of a survivable defect, we would accept the baby and help him or her grow into the best person possible.

I gave birth when I was 44 years old. Our child is 9 years old now, healthy and normal. Since preschool days, she has been a kind, insightful person who accepts other people as they present themselves. She has no patience with the concept of looking down on others for petty reasons—I hope that attitude will persist throughout her life. Perhaps for this reason, she accepts my seizures and occasional other odd behaviors in the context of my neurological disorder.

Our child has admonished us more than once: "Maman, you and Dad are like children!" It's true. My husband and I snipe at each other over matters so ridiculous that he and I laugh at ourselves. For example, there is the "car window fight": open (that's me), or closed (him). Then there's the "go this way fight": "Now you'll have to stop for lights" (me); "Your way is too long" (him). And the very popular " 'I-told-you-so' fight": (that's both of us). Those fights have invariable scripts; they're like *no* plays of the absurd. Not *kyogen* interludes, for we're deadly serious while we're acting our roles, and we sound as though the issues are ones of life and death weightiness. On the other hand, we never disagree on important matters. On important matters, we think alike.

Personal Stories

Can I rightly complain about my husband being overprotective? At one time, he may have been, but I can't recall the reasons behind this impression. Maybe it was because he was troubled by my seizures in the beginning, since he wasn't sure how to cope with them. He learned, though, and is no longer overprotective.

Our life together doesn't deny the seizures; neither does it revolve around them. What keeps us strong is what keeps any decent marriage strong: sharing interests, enjoying each other's company and achievements, and never taking each other for granted. Too, we've walked hand-in-hand past milestones: the birth of a child, the death of a parent, the unexpected illness and death of a close friend, and the treatment and recovery from an illness that threatened my husband's life.

My husband and I aren't identical. I'll never be a sailor; he'll never be captivated by cookbooks. He'll always be gregarious; I'll always be reticent. He's on the squeamish side; I'm not. But in matters of ethics and the like, we're the same. We're both somewhat eccentric, which is, no doubt, a much better situation than a partnership containing only one eccentric member.

For the past several years, the field I've been working in has proved a wise choice for me. I've been able to work regular hours during the day, get the chance to use my skills and art talent, and even have the time to continue my vocation as a working fine artist.

I have a short commute. I do hold a valid license, but I don't like to tempt fate by driving more than relatively short distances because my reaction time is slow and I can become confused easily while driving.

I hope that what I've written will be helpful. Anyone with temporal lobe epilepsy knows firsthand about the suffering that the disorder brings, and has felt the intensity of moods that it causes. I treat those aspects of my life as givens and can say that even against that backdrop, it has still been possible for me to lead a good life with friendship, love, and accomplishments to rejoice in.

For all the pain, I'd still rather be the way I am. I believe firmly that having epilepsy and dealing with it have made me a stronger, more resilient, more insightful person than I would have ever been otherwise.

3

(Age 60) I have had temporal lobe epilepsy for about 5 or 6 years. I was at work at a department store when a manager confronted me. He claimed I was not doing my job. I blew up at him and I had my very first seizure. Since then, I usually have a seizure whenever I get nervous or stressed out.

When I first go into a seizure, I get a strong smell of ammonia and my face and neck turn beet red. Then I black out and get a faraway look. I can hear others but I cannot answer them.

When I come out of it, I feel like I just did 8 hours of work! I'm very tired.

4

(Age 35) I am a survivor of sexual, physical, and emotional abuse. Perhaps the abuse ultimately caused the car accident when I was 16 that led to the epilepsy. Perhaps not. What matters now is that I've got seizures, and epilepsy affects every part of my life.

I am a lesbian woman and have had a life partner for 6 years. By the time we met, I had been having seizures for many years but was not receiving treatment because, for most of this time, I did not know what they were.

I am not a person who likes to go to the doctor and I am wary of treatments and medications. But after many discussions with my partner and, ultimately, a seizure that caused loss of consciousness, I finally relented and went to a doctor to find out what was going on. I have now been on treatment for over 3 years.

When I was first diagnosed with epilepsy and put on medication, I felt incredible fatigue and needed to sleep several hours during the day. Yet, despite this, I did not want to believe that anything had changed. I had many fights with her about my independence and whether I could drive somewhere or go to a meeting that would entail a 112-mile trip. The last fight over this almost caused our breakup, but I finally realized I was incapable of going on as if nothing was different. As a result, I began to take better care of myself.

Even though I have learned to deal with not driving, my independence seems nonexistent and my loss of control is enormous. Relying on others has always been difficult. My friends and family have pitched in to help, and I am very grateful for that. My jobs entail a lot of driving and travel throughout the state, and I could not do it without them and public transportation (bus and train).

My cognitive functioning can be seriously affected by changes in medication dosages. My speech, thought processes, and word finding, to name a few, are all compromised by medication. My visual fields and balance can be thrown out of whack, too. My partner has been supportive through all my mental and cognitive changes.

My intimate life with my partner has been affected greatly as well. My sexual drive at times can be nonexistent due to the medications' side effects. We try to figure out how to be close and maintain this closeness even at times that do not include sexual intimacy.

This can be hard to do, but there are many levels of intimacy, and we enjoy each other in many different ways. We continue to be strong in our relationship.

We have had an incredible amount of stress and anxiety in dealing with my epilepsy. At times I feel like a failure, not able to be present and participate fully as a partner in our day-to-day life together. These are powerful feelings and often batter my self-respect. But we do things on the good days, and when I need to take a nap, I do just that without argument or issue.

Recently, we have had to deal with even more in our relationship. My partner was diagnosed with multiple sclerosis. She had an incredible flare-up that could be barely managed with steroids. She lost sight in her left eye, and a tremendous amount of her physical ability was compromised. Unfortunately, because of insurance delays, she had to wait many months after the diagnosis to receive pharmacologic treatment.

After she became so sick, I was called on to be her driver during very difficult times. Our stress levels were extremely high and our relationship was pushed and pulled to the max. But through it all, we prevailed and held onto our love and commitment to each other. My partner's multiple sclerosis symptoms have now decreased, and she is able to walk and drive again.

In the beginning, my friends had a hard time with my epilepsy. They were afraid and did not know how to handle it. I felt distanced from them. I spoke with each friend individually to talk about his or her fears and to ask for support. All have responded positively and have supported my partner and me as we deal with my epilepsy and her multiple sclerosis.

My family had a difficult time accepting my epilepsy as well. Even when I had a seizure at their home, my parents were frightened and expected everything to be "all right" when I came out of it. When I was not "all right," they did not know how to respond. They later called me many times to see how I was feeling and if every-thing was "back to normal." Their perception of "normal" did not match mine. When I could not give them the answer they needed to hear, I was given replies of "you'll be just fine" or "you're making too much of it." I felt an incredible amount of stress from them to be "OK." When I wasn't "OK," I didn't want to talk with them about it. I distanced myself emotionally.

I reentered counseling after more than a 5-year absence. I worked on coming to terms with all the pent up emotions I had with epilepsy, my relationship with my partner, dealing with her multiple sclerosis, dealing with family, and working through my depression.

When I began therapy again, I felt less than a person—less competent and less independent. Therapy has helped me regain some of that. I also asked my family and parents to attend a local epilepsy conference, since there were many topics for families being presented. My mother went, and she did get something out of it. She connected with the other family members and parents.

My workplace has been very understanding and flexible. I have been able to defer some work-related travel and do teleconferences as needed. Still, I do attempt to get to my monthly meetings as much as possible with help from friends and family. I still am responsible for a full caseload, and I put pressure on myself to maintain the same work quality as before. Medication side effects have played a big role in decreasing my work output, but I still make the effort to achieve a high standard of work. My work ethic is strong and my employer knows this.

I know that epilepsy is something I have to live with. I hope that my situation stabilizes so I can regain the enjoyment of life and participate in various activities I used to be involved in. Conquering the fatigue, maintaining my independence, and continuing my relationships are the goals I am striving for now and for the future.

5

(Age 31) I don't feel seizures have affected my relationships or menstrual functions. But because I have epilepsy, I have decided not to have children unless I plan ahead with the advice of my doctors and take precautions. I am now single, so this has not become a problem.

Sometimes a person who is unfamiliar with seizures may be frightened when they're told that someone they know has epilepsy. But usually, once they have asked questions and gotten the proper answers, they are no longer frightened. I have never felt that hiding my epilepsy from people was the best thing to do. Whenever I am in a relationship, I always tell the other person about my epilepsy. I explain how I act during a seizure and then explain what to do if I have one.

I don't feel that I have ever been turned away from anyone because I had epilepsy. If anything, I think the fact that I have put on weight has been my downfall at times.

The hardest part of having seizures is that I cannot drive. I am well known to the cab and bus companies in my town. So, once a year, to make myself feel well, I go on a great vacation. I figure that I'm spending the money I have saved in gas and car payments.

6

(Age 43) My daughter, Beth, started having seizures when she was 10. At first it was very devastating for her and for us. Over time, thanks to loving family members, relatives, and friends, we were all able to cope with her seizures.

As a child, Beth went to special schools. She now attends a place for adults with cognitive disabilities and is very happy there.

She can do quite a bit. She loves to go bowling and dancing and get together with her peers for other activities. Her social life is being with friends and relatives.

Beth is a happy and well-adjusted person who likes to be included in family gatherings and go out to dinner. She is very pleasant to have around.

7

(Age 43) I am a single woman of 43 years. Has epilepsy played a role in my life as a female in this world? I try not to think about it. Even so, while I don't believe epilepsy is the reason I have not found a life partner or become a mother, I do think it has shaped my life.

I always felt it necessary to explain my seizure disorder to my date, lest I have a seizure in front of the man, leaving him scared, confused, and helpless. Because my seizures only occur during sleep, this usually meant waiting until the relationship had advanced to the stage of sexual intimacy, unless the subject had come up earlier.

Needless to say, there is always a risk that a man will be unable to tolerate the impact that epilepsy might have on a relationship. Whenever I disclosed my epilepsy, I faced a variety of responses from complete acceptance to fear. I have been with men who admire my strength in coping well with a difficult problem. Then there are other men who shied away from me after hearing this news. One man responded by saying he knew what to expect because he had once dated a woman with schizophrenia. I never heard from him again.

Motherhood is a story not unrelated to finding a man. To become pregnant, I would first have to adjust my medication. I am sure that this adjustment would be guided by the current wisdom of the field. But I would still be worried, justifiably so, that my life and my abilities to drive and to work would be put in jeopardy because of the possibility that a seizure could occur during the daytime. My wish to be a mother has always come second to my heartfelt need to take care of myself. Becoming pregnant is a risk that I am personally not willing to take.

Since our culture attaches so much meaning to motherhood as a symbol of womanhood, it's been important for me to find meaning in my life as a woman despite not being a mother. I am pleased to have arrived at a point of self-acceptance with the knowledge that I have the *capability* to be a good mother and can find other ways in my life of mothering.

8

(Age 36) When I was 15 years old, a Portuguese man-of-war poisoned me. The sting was so painful that I was rushed to an emergency ward, where I was given a cortisone shot. An allergic reaction to this medication triggered off various recurring neurological symptoms, such as twitching and shaking, and loss of concentration. Eventually, after numerous CT scans and EEGs, it was determined that I had a seizure disorder.

As a young person, I was traumatized by this experience and the episodic symptoms. I was taken out of school and had home tutoring. I was even taken across the western part of the country in the hope of being detoxified.

My condition affected me socially during my teenage years. Dating was difficult. Attending a small private school helped me to slowly develop friendships once again. I would be asked why I had gone to private school, and why after that I went to college and lived at home.

I am very grateful that I have a caring and supportive family that stood by me during this period in my life. I feel that, as a result, I was able to become independent. I now have a teaching position that I enjoy and have nearly completed two graduate degree programs.

When I was in my early 20s, I was told that seizure medications could cause serious problems for an unborn child. I was so frightened by this information that I did not want to enter into a serious relationship. But when I was 34, I met a wonderful man. As our relationship developed, I told him about my accident, the seizure disorder, and the possible effects of my medication on an unborn child. He was very supportive of me, for which I am grateful.

We have now been happily married for 1 year. My neurologist referred me to another epilepsy specialist, who supports and helps women with seizure disorders who would like to become pregnant.

Under my doctor's direction, I have been decreasing my medication for a month now and hope to be completely off in another month. I faithfully practice stress reduction techniques for relieving stress as well as reducing headaches. I am also exercising at least 45 to 50 minutes a day. I am taking folic acid and beginning to feel positive and optimistic, hoping for the best.

One has to be grateful for having a supportive family and spouse and trustworthy doctors.

9

(Age 53) When I became pregnant with my first child, I started to feel odd sensations. Sometimes I had lightheadedness; other times I had the feeling that butterflies were swarming inside my stomach. Throughout my pregnancy, these unfamiliar feelings would occasionally occur. I delivered a healthy baby weighing 8 lb without any problem.

Shortly after my child was born, I had my first grand mal seizure and was diagnosed with epilepsy. I then started taking anticonvulsant medications. Over the course of 5 years, I delivered two more children with no problems during either pregnancy or delivery, even while taking medications. I am now perimenopausal and experience more seizures than I did in the past, probably due to the hormonal imbalance that eventually occurs in all of us women.

I do not feel that my epilepsy caused many problems during my years of dating. I was honest and open in describing what may possibly occur, and what to do if I had a seizure. Most importantly, I said not to be afraid. I stressed that it was OK to be concerned, but to remember that I would be all right after a seizure. During my years of marriage, my husband would help me when the need arose. The children grew up with their mother having "this problem" and did not allow it to interfere with their lives. I explained the necessities to them so that they would not be scared and would know what to do. They are now living accomplished lives of their own and love me and are proud of me.

Over the years, having epilepsy did affect my emotional security and confidence, but I wanted to live as normal a life as possible. The first most important thing I did was to *accept* my diagnosis and be proud of who I was.

With my desire and determination, I have continued to live my life. Working a full-time job (after explaining about my seizures to my supervisor, a cot was made available in my time of need) has helped me regain my independence and socialize with my friends with full enjoyment.

Yes, at times life has been rough, but we can do it. All we need is *desire* and *determination* in order to make the decision to succeed.

And we need *faith* to reach our destination.

10

(Age 21) I was not diagnosed with epilepsy until I was a senior in high school. I am now 21 years old, so I have dealt with this for only 3 years now. At first, it was a little scary to hear the neurologist say "You have epilepsy," but it was even more frustrating before the diagnosis was made because my family and I had no idea what was wrong with me. At least having a diagnosis brought a bit of relief.

At times I consider myself very lucky. There are so many people who have epilepsy that is more severe than mine. I have experienced a grand mal seizure; however, I have no memory of it. My mother is the one that has the not-so-pleasant honor of being able to recall the scene. I consider myself lucky because on a regular day-to-day basis, I just pop pills.

Are there frustrating moments? Oh yes! Sometimes it can be a pain to remember to take my pills twice a day, every day. Or, if I forget them, to turn around and go back and get them; or to pack extra pills when I am on vacation. Being reminded by loving and concerned parents is nice sometimes, but overbearing at other times.

Since the diagnosis, I have been through two different relation-ships in which my significant other asked me about the seizures. I can understand why, but sometimes it can damage the ego. I am in a relationship now—my boyfriend reminds me to take my pills, tells me to get to bed early, and is totally accepting of my condition.

The hardest aspect, I would have to say, is not being able to drive for 6 months after every seizure. Telling a college student to get to bed early, not to drink alcohol, and to remain as unstressed as possible is one thing, but to then tell them they cannot drive is another. I am a pretty independent person, so for me to have to ask someone to take me somewhere is a hard thing to do and wears thin pretty fast. I can honestly say it is the one thing I hate the most about having epilepsy.

I always find that the easiest way to deal with a situation such as mine is to look at it positively. My case is not severe by any means, and as of now it is controlled. I asked about having children and was told that most healthy women have a 96 percent chance of having a healthy baby, and that I have a 94 percent chance.

Everyone has something they must deal with in life and mine happens to be very manageable. I have a great life and a wonderful future to look forward to.

11

(Age 33) I am a 33-year-old female with epilepsy. I was diagnosed at the age of 19, as a young college student. I don't feel I was treated differently than anyone else back then.

I met my husband the day after my first seizure. I did not take my epilepsy very seriously then. Nor did he, until after we were married and he started witnessing seizures. That scared him.

I truly started feeling that I was different after I married my husband. Both his parents and mine started mentioning to me that they did not think we should have children. They were afraid of what would happen if I should have a seizure while pregnant or that I would have a child with epilepsy or even birth defects.

I had doctors who never totally reassured me about these things. We started to look into the possibility of adopting. I had several friends and family members who had adopted children and told us stories about how difficult it would be for us to adopt because of my epilepsy—we would not be "choice" parents.

The notion of being parents began to sound hopeless for us. I saw many different neurologists before I found one who actually supported our decision to have children. And I went to eight different gynecologists before I found one who would even work with my neurologist and me. One told me he could not agree to take care of me through the pregnancy if I stayed on the same seizure medication.

My husband and I have been married for 9 years. We have not had children yet. We have never used birth control, but my cycle has not been normal in years. I have read that this may be caused by my seizure medication, but I have also read many conflicting reports. Each day I have to take twenty doses of my seizure medication, 4 mg of folic acid, vitamins, and other pills for fertility. Just taking them is a problem because it is so time consuming. Not to mention the fact that the seizure medication is in capsule form, and the plastic sometimes makes me sick to my stomach.

Since the day I was diagnosed with epilepsy, my mother has treated me like the weakest of her six children. She is a very strong and independent woman, but she is always afraid something is going to happen to me. My father told me never to reveal my epilepsy to anyone. I am not quite sure if he is ashamed by my epilepsy or if he thinks I may be treated differently if I tell other people.

My husband is *very* protective; he asks me not to drive long distances because he is terrified that I might have a seizure while driving, especially at night. We have had a few arguments over this, since my family lives 200 miles from me. But then I come to my senses and wait until he can travel with me. It is difficult to truly feel independent when I have to rely on my husband like this.

Because insufficient sleep could lead to my seizures, my sleep habits have changed dramatically. My husband loves to stay up late at night, but I have to go to bed early. I used to be a very social person, but now I have a difficult time going out with our friends because they like to stay out late. We are always the first to leave. It's not a big problem, but it makes me feel a little guilty.

Overall, epilepsy has not become a problem in my life but something that I have to add to my routine. Now that I know my limits, I can control my seizures by taking care of myself and taking my medication. My seizures have not changed the way I feel deep down about myself in the least.

12

(Age 27) My first seizure was at age 14. It was at school in front of many classmates and teachers. Going back to school a few days later was tough, but I learned from the very beginning how to deal with other people who possibly viewed me as different. To my surprise, I arrived to find that everyone treated me very much the same. They all seemed to have some knowledge and understanding about epilepsy. I assume that the teachers must have addressed it while I was absent.

My seizures from that point on were few and far between, but even now, after being seizure-free for almost 5 years, not a day goes by that I don't wonder whether I will have one. Where will it happen? Will I be around strangers? Will I be safe?

Fortunately, epilepsy never really affected my family life—at least not from my perspective. Maybe my parents were stressed over it, but it never showed. I saw that they were confident in my ability to continue living my life just as anyone else would, and that gave me confidence.

It wasn't until my husband and I began discussing the possibility of having children that my epilepsy became a concern. I was 24. We knew we would have to do some planning and went to see the neurologist who had been treating me for the past 10 years.

I always knew that seizure medications could possibly affect a fetus, but nothing could have prepared us for the news we got. We were told that the particular medication I was taking carried an extremely high risk for causing neural tube defects in a developing fetus as well as heart defects. I was strongly advised not to get pregnant, and if I became pregnant, to terminate it.

He did give me the option to change my medication to something else that had a lower risk. I felt like I was being forced to choose what kind of health problems would affect my child, as if having a healthy normal child was completely out of the question. I held my breath until we got in the car and then cried for what seemed like days. I had no idea how much I wanted children until that day.

A year later, after much consideration, I decided to go ahead and try a new medication. I had a severe allergic reaction to it and ended up semiconscious in the emergency room. After 12 years of living with epilepsy and being virtually unaffected by it, I now felt that having the family I always wanted was an unreachable goal. I quickly convinced myself that children were not important and that there were other things I could do in life. That is how I protected myself from deep sadness over the thought of not having children.

It took about a month before I was back to normal physically. In that time, my mother had obtained the number for a new epilepsy specialist. She had heard about this doctor's program for women with epilepsy. I made an appointment.

The night before my appointment, I found out I was pregnant. I felt so irresponsible, knowing what things could happen to this baby because of my condition. Instead of going to my appointment with the new doctor, I almost headed for the nearest abortion clinic. Thankfully, my husband and parents assured me it would all be fine and encouraged me to see what the new neurologist had to say.

Well, what she said saved my daughter's life—literally. It turned out the risks and concerns of my pregnancy weren't much higher than usual. Yes, there were some precautions we had to take, but there was no reason to believe that I couldn't have a healthy child. I am so grateful to have met this doctor and her staff, and grateful for their knowledge of epilepsy and pregnancy.

Every time I look at my daughter, I can't believe I almost gave her up before even getting to meet her. She is beautiful and perfect in every way. Giving birth to her was an amazing experience, and now I have the confidence to do it again.

13

(Age 49) My seizure activity began very slowly 10 years ago. At the time, I had no idea what I was experiencing. I was working in the office of the neighborhood school where my two boys had gone. I found that my consciousness was suddenly taken over by a familiar thought. I went into a "trance" for 30 seconds. Afterward, my brain didn't function 100 percent, and I felt like I was on auxiliary power. I became embarrassed and wanted to go home, which I did.

Due to unrelated reasons, I left the job and started working for a family member who happens to be a state senator. He was very compassionate but wanted me to solve my problem. My problem was then diagnosed as epilepsy.

It became very stressful and embarrassing to have seizures—particularly once at work, when I went down to the floor like I had fainted but was apparently shaking, and once while driving. Even the slight seizures that I experienced, while not big problems, were inconveniences while I was working.

I was forced to take action. I now knew that I could no longer avoid medication. My brother also suffers from seizures, though his are much more severe. He had been on many different medications and had experienced problems. Because of that, my husband and I were both very skeptical about the side effects of such medications.

However, since being put on seizure medication 7 months ago, I have not experienced any seizures at all. This medication was put to the test when I lost a very dear friend and did not have any breakthrough seizures.

14

(Age 16) One Saturday last September is a day I will never forget. I was getting ready to go to work with my dad in our family business, when suddenly I blacked out and collapsed. I barely remember trying to regain consciousness and struggling to pull myself up. A while later, my dad found me lying in the middle of the floor and thought I had fallen asleep there. He walked me back to bed and later had me get ready to leave. I was very tired and slept most of the day.

I didn't think much about what had happened at the time, but it happened a second time 1 month later. My dad said it was about 5:00 a.m. when he and mom were startled awake by a loud noise. He said they ran into my bedroom and turned on the light, only to find me piled up in the corner of the room on the floor with my neck twisted in an awkward position against the wall. They both thought I had fallen and broken my neck. My parents said they carefully pulled me away from the wall and worked with me for what seemed like forever but was probably more like 10 to 15 minutes. They said I was unconscious and then started to shake violently.

As my mom called 911, my dad and sister attempted to give me mouth-to-mouth resuscitation. My parents say that the worst time of their lives was when my dad was holding me in his arms and all of a sudden I quit shaking and went limp. They say they almost panicked when my eyes rolled back into my head and I appeared to stop breathing.

About that time, three paramedics arrived and said I most likely had a seizure. A few moments later, I made a breathing noise and slowly began to regain consciousness. Dad said that was the most joyous moment he could remember. The paramedics suggested that my parents let me rest for a while, as I was very exhausted.

That afternoon my mom and dad took me to the doctor. She did an EKG and also referred me to a neurologist. I saw the neurologist later that week. She gave me a prescription for an antiseizure medicine. After taking it for about two weeks, I got real sick. I had a fever and broke out with a bad rash. Right away I went back to the doctor and she prescribed a different antiseizure medication, which I am still taking. I have to admit I was getting pretty sick of going to the doctor, but I did get to miss school a couple of times.

My doctor scheduled me for more EKGs and a sleep-deprived EEG, as well as lab tests. The sleep-deprived EEG, for me, was the worst test that I had to prepare for. My mom had the "fun" job of keeping me awake all night. We went to the movies at 2:00 a.m. and went to a restaurant around 4:00 a.m. It was very weird.

Probably the worst test to actually go through was the MRI. I could not stand being in such a tight place for such a long time. I pray that I will *never* have to have another one as long as I live.

After I had been on the second seizure medication for a while, I started to notice that some of my hair was coming out. I told my doctor about this, and she gave me a bunch of vitamins that I must now take. I feel sort of funny because I have to take four different types of medications each morning, for a total of ten pills a day. But ever since I started taking the vitamins, I have not had to worry about my hair falling out anymore.

For several months, it was very hard for me. I got to where I was scared to get up in the middle of the night for fear of having another seizure. For about 2 weeks I traded beds with my dad so I could sleep with my mom. Now I am not nearly as scared of having another seizure as I was.

Once in a while I do worry about having another seizure. I'm worried that I might have one while I'm out in public, with my friends, or even worse, while driving! I find it hard sometimes to remember to take my medicine, especially since I have to take it three times a day. I feel bad because I get irritated with my parents for asking me if I've taken my medicine. I do, however, appreciate them greatly and how much they show their concern for me. I also find myself wondering if I'm going to be taking antiseizure medicine for the rest of my life. I often question if I would ever have another seizure if I were to stop taking my medicine, but I don't think I have the nerve to try.

I know that it was through the help of my parents and God that I'm doing just fine now.

15

(Age 55) After 20 years of being free of seizures, they came back with a vengeance.

Here I was—beginning the empty nest syndrome, showing signs of menopause, and starting a new job. The immediate effect of the return of seizures was the loss of my independence. Since I can't drive now, I have to inconvenience my family or friends for rides.

I find it very difficult to ask, even though they are very willing and reassure me that it is no problem. The funny thing is, if the situation were reversed, I would gladly put myself out for them.

I really don't know when the seizures are about to happen, although I think I'm getting better adjusted to that. But I just don't want to wimp out. I feel I should be able to tough it out. My family can predict the onset of a seizure. I'll often snap at them that I'm all right. They have never come out and said it, but I feel they think it's my fault and that I should be able to control the seizures. My husband realizes I want to do things for myself and will often just let me work it out on my own.

Most people accept my condition as long as I don't use the word "epilepsy." But stereotypes are still out there, like the hairdresser who said women with epilepsy couldn't have children. Well, I have four healthy, bright children.

When I first went to the medical center, I felt that the doctors there should have been able to give me answers and control my seizures completely, but there weren't any answers or cures. There were only more questions and trials of new medications.

Now my fear is that because we are concentrating on the seizures, there may be other things going wrong with my body that we are ignoring. I do keep contact with my primary care physician, but I know his first perception is "seizures and overweight." Sometimes I feel if I could lose the weight, everything would be fine. I hate how I look but do everything to sabotage myself.

My right to work as a teacher is protected under the Americans with Disabilities Act. But how would you feel knowing your child's teacher had a seizure in front of her second grade class? How do you think I feel after awakening in the hospital and realizing this? The first time, I was embarrassed. I felt I had let everyone down and was ready to resign and stay home. My family and friends encouraged me to lessen the job stress by working half-time. That strategy, along with new medication, has seemed to help.

16

(Age 43) I mostly still have my seizures once a month. This is despite the fact that I've had my ovaries and uterus removed—and I don't have any more actual periods. Even so, when the date comes up that I would have usually expected my period, I still have seizures!

It's very hard trying to get a job when you have seizures. If you have one on the job, they send you home. I was out of work for 4 weeks and was put on another medicine and felt better. I was told to go back to work, but that they would only accept me 3 days a week. I couldn't go back full time like I used to do work.

It's a terrible feeling, having seizures.

17

(Age 47) I developed epilepsy at the age of 14. From the very beginning, my parents and siblings were always very caring and supportive, but they did not allow me to use seizures as an excuse. As a result, epilepsy has not affected my family relationships or my friendships because I have not let it. I always let people know I have epilepsy, but do not use it as a "pity me" tool.

When I was 24 years old, I moved to a different state in order to gain my independence. I was in between jobs, and my best friend suggested the move. It was the best thing I ever did. Until that time, I was very dependent on my parents and needed to get that far away so that I couldn't run home every time I had a seizure or something went wrong.

After 4 years, I decided to move back. By that time, I had developed my independence, and though I was still actively seizing, I found a job, moved into the city, and was able to maintain my independence. Staying financially stable was rough due to the large doctor bills and costs of medication. However, I did not let this get me down—I just kept on barreling along.

Around 4 years ago, it was discovered that my seizures were hormonally based. I was put on progesterone and became seizure-free. Six months ago, I was started on estrogen because I was starting menopause. Unfortunately, the initial dosage was too high and 1 month later I had six seizures in 48 hours. The dosage of estrogen was lowered immediately, and I have not had any seizures since that time.

To sum things up: my main message to other women, whether they have been seizing for many years or have just developed epilepsy, is you must not let seizures affect your life! After having a seizure, you just have to "pick yourself up, dust yourself off, and start all over again!"

Do not let the fact you have epilepsy stand in your way of becoming independent, developing a romantic relationship, holding a job, or being active in the community. Life's too short.

18

(Age 39) I have seizures at least once a month due to my period. The seizure comes either at the beginning of the cycle or at the end. I hate having seizures because they affect my work. When I have a seizure, I have to take a day off because of the aftereffects. I have tried different medications, but none has really worked for me. My case is a difficult one.

I would love to have children, but I don't think my body could take it. I am also on several seizure medications, which would make it hard.

I wish I didn't have seizures because I know I can die from one. If fact, because I have nearly died five times, I am very happy to be alive! I am happy to be working and to be a part of society and enjoying it, and being a part of something that I love to do.

I try really hard every day, and it's not easy for me. Some days are better than others. I feel very sad when I have to go through a seizure. I wish people would understand my epilepsy, but not everyone does. Where I work, though, most people understand and are very willing to help me out. I thank them for that.

I wish I had a higher paying job, but I don't. Even so, I am doing fine, and that's all that really matters. I also have a very supportive family, which really counts. Any time that I need them, they are there for me to give me advice. I love them all for it.

But I must say that women with epilepsy go through a lot every day—and it's not easy.

19

(Age 45) As a child, I was put on a seizure medication that can cause hair to grow all over. I'm told that my first response to having this happen to me was to run to my mother and say, "Look at my arms, they're all hairy!" I don't remember this, but I do remember going to school and being called names like "monkey" and excluded from groups of children because they thought I looked like a "boy." I always thought that the cruelest thing a teenager can say to a peer is "You look like a man because you have a mustache." I suppose other events like this kept coming up, but I eventually learned to cope with it.

I know my first tonic-clonic seizure was related to hormonal changes, because it happened along with my first cycle (and about that time of month every month afterwards).

I was interested in school dances and went to a number of them, but it never failed—I always had a seizure. Sometimes I thought other boys didn't ask me to dance because I would usually have a seizure while dancing. This never stopped me, though! To this day, I still keep on dancing or doing my thing.

I know a lot of damage has been done by one of the seizure medications I have taken. I feel as though I lost many years of my life, acting—as my brother puts it—"like a zombie." I was in a special school for children with learning disabilities from grades 7 to 9. Then I had a private tutor until I graduated high school.

Life with epilepsy as a child, teenager, family member, and woman has not been easy. I usually try to forget about it. I have always lived like this. I carry identification and insurance cards just in case I have a seizure, but I go on with my life the way I want to. Yes, doing this can bring dangers. I've had many sutures because of falls off of bicycles, but I've also had sutures to stitch up injuries that happened while food shopping. I figure it's all a matter of timing. Why sit at home and wait for a seizure when there is so much to do today?

As far as family relationships are concerned, I was always very close to my aunt and uncle. But when I started having seizures, my aunt never wanted to be alone in the house with me. It took me years to find out it was because she was afraid I might have a seizure.

Someone else in my family used to think I might drop or injure her baby and would never let me hold her children. Now that my seizures are under control, she still offends me by asking every time she sees me, "How long has it been since your last seizure?" If she does it again, I may sever my relationship with her.

Just because you have epilepsy does not mean you can't have a nice boyfriend or husband, children, a good job, a nice home, and anything else you may dream of. It just means you have to work a little harder to get them. I now have a part-time job, and my seizures are under control. I have a wonderful partner, and we are working on a house for the future.

Yes, my epilepsy will always be there; I only hope that I will always be around to help people understand epilepsy.

20

(Age 42) My seizures developed after I had been involved in two automobile accidents. While it took me a while to fully understand what was happening to me, it was clear from the beginning that other people didn't know how to deal with my seizures or the other complication that I had, postconcussion syndrome. As a result, from the start I felt shame, in addition to confusion, about what was wrong with me.

Not being able to drive left me feeling isolated. The loss of independence made me feel very dependent on others and angry.

My husband and I had to choose not to have children because of my age, the fear that the hormonal changes of pregnancy would cause an increase in seizures, and the fact that I couldn't drive. Somehow, I don't always fit in with my friends who have their own families. Holidays can be tough when spent visiting these friends and their children, particularly when we receive photos of their families.

There is another side to my seizures. Things happen for a reason, and I have always looked upon my seizures as a gift on some level. Because of this attitude, I have come to know myself better—to slow down, take better care of myself, make better lifestyle choices, seek out jobs with less stress, and have faith that people can help and want to support you. I have learned to pass over those who can't or won't help. I have become more patient and trusting, even through the difficult times.

I try hard to enjoy and simplify life. I have been more supportive and understanding of the limitations of people whether or not they have disabilities. I look at the person, not his or her problem.

I get up every day knowing that I have seizures, but also with the hope that this may be the last day I will have a seizure. I will never lose faith that day will come.

21

(Age 29) I met my husband when I was 19 years old, which is, ironically, the same age when I began to have seizures (a running joke between us). In fact, I had my first *big* (generalized) seizure while sleeping at his dorm. He was very moved by the whole experience, as he had never witnessed one.

Over the past 10 years, I actually feel that my disorder has been a bond between us. I'm certainly not saying that I wouldn't love to never have another seizure again, but it's nice to have the support that I have. My husband's view on living with my seizures is "Of course it's scary at times, but I actually think it's *cool*: it makes you unique, it's the only way I have known you."

With respect to my family and friends, I would say that they seem almost fascinated to hear about seizures. Typically, people don't want to ask how my seizures are doing. But if I offer the information first, they seem to have endless questions! "What's it like?" "Can you feel them?" "Does it hurt?" And of course, "What should I do if you have one while you are with me?"

I have found that being open and honest about my seizures is very helpful. Besides, the way I look at it, I didn't do anything wrong to get epilepsy, so why should I hide it? When you are open about it, the message that you send to others is "I am comfortable with my epilepsy, so you can learn about my seizures from me. You don't have to ask other people."

Dealing with my seizures in my professional life is probably the most difficult thing for me. I am a school psychologist, so I work with young children every day. My biggest fear is that I will have a seizure in front of one of my students and scare him or her. Luckily, the children probably wouldn't notice a seizure because I just stare off.

With my colleagues, however, I have been very open from day one. I announced my disorder in the lunchroom after only being at my job for a week or two. Again, people were fascinated. I sometimes feel that people think that you can't be a professional if you have epilepsy. I have had seizures in front of the school staff, but because everyone knew about it, there was only a moderate "oh my God" response. I must admit that my popularity soared! Everyone is curious about things they witness yet don't understand.

Being that I am approaching the age at which I would like to start a family, I have new fears. My (female) doctor does a wonderful job explaining the concerns that I should and shouldn't have. For example, prior to meeting my doctor, I thought that I wouldn't even be able to breast-feed my baby. I'm disappointed that I can't just "get pregnant." Because of the medication issues, I must sit and truly plan my pregnancies, and I'm sure I will spend 9 months of complete worrying if all will be okay.

Then again, what woman doesn't?

22

(Age 39) In the beginning, seizures for me were something of a mystery. I never knew that I was having them. I wasn't alone—it took doctors over 10 years to actually figure out that my "dream states" were seizures, not just something I was imagining.

My seizures were like dreams that happened while I was awake. Staring off at something became a "normal" thing for me. Shaking my head to come back to reality was like waking myself up from the dream. The only problem was that when the "dream" ended, I felt lost, as if time had gone by and I was stuck somewhere back a few minutes.

After suffering my one and only grand mal seizure, everything changed. My seizures became more violent, and my world soon turned upside down. People would leave the room during my seizures. No one would help me. When I needed to talk about them, no one would listen with open ears, let alone a caring heart. No one understood.

I went out on dates, but if I had a seizure, it would be the last date with that person. No one wanted to date the girl with the "problem."

Eventually, I did get married. The man I married had a hard time dealing with the seizures, although he never said so. He would stand off at a distance and watch while I had one. I doubt he ever realized what was going on.

Then I underwent brain surgery to control my seizures. It changed my life. After my surgery, I was seizure-free, but my world came crashing in. My husband still expected me to be the same person, someone who needed to lean on him for everything. He expected our sex life to be the same, and he wanted it immediately after the surgery. In my mind, there were other things to deal with first.

Personal Stories

I became independent and more sure of myself and who I was. I had goals to reach and dreams to fulfill. My husband felt he should be top priority. Our marriage, for these many reasons, fell apart.

Life moved on for me. I was taken off medications a few years down the road, and to this day I am still seizure-free. I am lucky . . . and blessed . . . and grateful!

My family and I went through some very hard times after my surgery. I had changed emotionally—so much so, that for several years there were few letters and even fewer calls between us. It was very hard for my mother to adjust to hearing that her daughter had epilepsy. I had been labeled, and that label in her view had left me "bruised"—like a bruised peach—for life.

Everyone wanted me to remain the same; only trouble was, after the surgery, I was not the same. I wanted what everyone else had—independence. We had fights, exchanged words, and let anger win out. My relationships with everyone became so strained that it was hard to talk to anyone. It was as if no one understood or knew me anymore—not even me at times—even though for the first time in years, I was actually free of seizures.

Friendships were hard hit at times, but my true friends never left my side. They may not have understood the changes that happened during my years of seizures and the years following the surgery, but they stuck with me, offered me hope, compassion, love, and understanding. I could not have asked for anything more.

When I had my surgery done, I thought, "I'm no longer epileptic!" I learned that the diagnosis never goes away. Oh, I may be seizure-free and off medication, but no one can promise me that the seizures will never return. No one can give that kind of a guarantee, so I live my life to the fullest. I strive to get the most out of each day that I am seizure-free. In many ways, I celebrate each day that I can be myself, without fearing what may or may not happen somewhere down the road.

Epilepsy in Our Lives

Nearly 10 years after my divorce, I met someone very special. I made a point to tell him *all* about my medical history, not expecting him to stick around. But he did—he accepted me for who I am. Seizure-free or not, it made no difference to him. We were married just over 3 years ago; less than 4 months after we met. Our marriage has had its rough times now and then, but we hold on to each other. No matter what medical problems have come or have yet to come, we rely on each other for support and encouragement.

I was always afraid I would never have a chance to have a family of my own. After suffering three miscarriages, I was, along with my husband, ready to accept the possibility of just the two of us together for the rest of our lives. But we were surprised last year to learn we were going to be parents. This time we were blessed, for we have a beautiful, healthy daughter.

There are people who say that epilepsy is a lifetime problem. Or that epilepsy is a disease. It's neither. Epilepsy is a medical condition. When diagnosed correctly, and followed closely by your doctor, you can still lead a rewarding life, even if you continue to have seizures. How? Don't let what other people say or feel keep you from being who you want to be. Don't let life pass you by because you are afraid to try something new. Take time to enjoy life, even if it's life in between seizures. Follow your doctor's advice, even if you don't like it—it can make a positive difference in your life.

Don't be afraid to share your medical history with someone. Sometimes being honest about your problems with seizures can help that other person relax and deal with it better. And if you have trouble with friends or family accepting the fact you have epilepsy, try to understand where they are coming from. I know firsthand that it is not easy for others to accept, but talking about it with them *does* help, on *both* sides. Remind them that you are still you and that you love them, faults and all. Sometimes that is all they need to hear to know you are OK. Sometimes reassuring them helps them to reassure you that life does go on, even for someone with epilepsy.

Personal Stories

37

Yes, life does go on. It has gone on for me, and I am extremely happy that it has. I may have epilepsy, but epilepsy does not have me. Most importantly, I am a person who has accepted her epilepsy and has managed to go on with living. I am content and ready for whatever comes my way.

23

(Age 46) I have had epilepsy all my life, so I know what it is like to have seizures. In the beginning, it was hard for me because no one understood what epilepsy was, including me.

As I grew up and tried unsuccessfully to go to work, the seizures got worse. People still did not seem to understand. Even the doctors. I got married and became pregnant. The doctors did not give me any special instructions or guidance, even though they knew I had seizures. My daughter was born with a heart defect and now has attention-deficit disorder.

Several years later, I finally met a doctor who understood. He helped me out more than anyone. If it was not for him, I would not have had the epilepsy surgery, and I might still be convinced that my seizures were "all in my head," like so many people had tried to tell me my entire life.

24

(Age 62) Except for poor vision, I had always had very good health. Then, 10 years ago, I had my first seizure after a very emotionally traumatic experience. I am sure that there was a connection, because there is no epilepsy in my family, and I had never had a seizure before or any significant head injury of which I am aware. The upsetting event happened on a Friday, and my first seizure happened the following Sunday evening. It was a very frightening experience.

I was brought to the emergency room, given medication, and had various tests. The scariest test was the MRI. Fortunately, I am not claustrophobic, so I managed quite well by counting the "bangs."

Despite the tests, there was no explanation for why I had the seizures. In fact, since then, there has never been, to the best of my knowledge, a clear understanding of why I have seizures. For several years, I took the same medication. Side effects were minimal, but I still had occasional seizures at night. I could tell if I had a grand mal seizure during the night because I was exhausted the next day, my cheeks were often chewed on the inside of my mouth, and my suitemate would usually be woken up because I made a vocalization noise just as the seizure was starting.

Generally these seizures did not disturb my work life or daily routine. Only my intimate friends knew of the problem.

But then certain side effects of the seizure medication became more pronounced, especially memory loss and lack of concentration. It was suggested that I try another medication. I agreed. It was while taking this new medication that I had my first daytime grand mal seizure. I then tried a third medication, only to go back to taking the original one for some reason. But then I developed nerve problems in my feet. They were not severe, but I was concerned.

Based on a suggestion from one of the nurses I knew, I changed to a new neurologist who had a very good reputation. She suggested that I switch to another drug because of its known effectiveness and low side effect profile. As I began the switch, the nerve problems in my feet decreased. But after the switch was complete, I started to fall randomly because of partial complex seizures. I fell in the kitchen, bathroom, while ironing, in church, at a craft fair, etc. Some things in the apartment, like a lamp, got broken without my knowing how it happened. This was terribly disconcerting. Fortunately, based on reports from friends, I tended to collapse rather gently during a seizure, as opposed to falling hard. Now I'm back to my old faithful medication, with some of the new one added in at a low dose to help control the numbness in my feet.

Although I know that there are many other medicinal choices I can make, I am both tired and fearful of experimenting. Even with my current medications, I occasionally lose my balance and fall during a seizure, but fortunately (at least to my knowledge), I've fallen when people were around to lower me down safely, until recently.

Perhaps I should add, before I continue, that I have no aura that I have been able to discern before a seizure. If I have a mild seizure that lasts only 20 or 30 seconds, then right after the seizure, I will continue doing what I was doing immediately before the seizure as if nothing happened. If I am in the middle of a conversation when this occurs, and someone suddenly asks me if I am feeling well, then I know I must have had a seizure. Otherwise, I would never know.

For the past several years, I have developed my own theory about why my seizures occur. I think that the seizures are connected to the hormone swings related to the onset of my menopause. I am presently 62 years old and am still perimenopausal. I know this is somewhat unusual, and it appears that there is no particular medical problem. Until recently, I thought that menopause had finally come and I was glad for the freedom. But, a couple months ago, I had another full period that was accompanied by several seizures over a couple of days. I started my period on a Tuesday morning and had a seizure that was close to a grand mal on Wednesday evening. Sometime the next day, I must have had other seizures, because someone helped me while I was falling up the stairs in front of a hospital library. I became aware that I was in a wheelchair and asked to be brought into the library to continue my work. Then, the next day while waiting for an elevator, I had another seizure and must have fallen very hard on the floor or against the elevator. I was brought to the emergency room. I remember nothing until the moment when a man asked me why I was lying on the floor. I said, "Oh, I was just tired." He said, "Thank goodness you didn't get tired in the middle of the street." I have no other recollection until I "woke up" in the emergency room. For the first time, I bruised myself quite badly during a seizure, forming black and blue marks that covered my whole left buttock and behind my left knee. It took several weeks for the bruises to clear up.

My suitemate says that when things like this happen, I initially try to make up a story and act as if all is normal. Sometimes I say things that do not make sense. I am not conscious of this at all.

It has been very difficult to deal with the unpredictability and total surprise of these seizures. For the first 5 or 6 years, they occurred primarily during the nighttime; thus, they were more acceptable and manageable. I sincerely hope that menopause will bring the end of these seizures.

Family and friends have been most supportive. My work as chaplain in a hospital did suffer, although the issue was never directly dealt with. It was both surprising and hurtful that a program that speaks of and supports "wounded healers" could deal with me in this way. Over time, and with the support of physicians, friends, and a center that focuses on the connection between the mind and body, I am coming to accept and deal with my situation.

I am still hoping that my menopause theory works out, but I am gradually preparing myself, with God's help, for any eventuality.

25

⌒

(Age 37) The "bad old days" would start with small complex partial seizures every few hours. I would still go to work. The seizures would consist of a feeling in the pit of my stomach that would travel up and get to the point that I would feel like I was going to throw up. I would swear I was going to throw up. I would hang my head over a barrel and tell everyone with such conviction that they would all believe me. Then the seizure was over. I never did throw up, not once.

Over time, my seizures began to increase in frequency and intensity until I was having grand mal seizures. When I lived alone, I would lie on my kitchen floor if I had a seizure because the kitchen was empty and so I couldn't hurt myself there. I also didn't want to ruin my mattress.

So I would lie there for a day or two. I would have several grand mals, and sometimes break a bone. I would pray the bad phase would hit on the weekend so I didn't miss work. After a day or so of grand mal seizures, the complex partial seizures would start to spread out in time and decrease in intensity.

By the next day, if I hadn't hurt myself, I could be back to work. I would still be having seizures and thinking I was going to throw up, but they never lasted too long. The whole thing, from the first hint of a seizure to the last eye twitch, took about a week. The only good thing was I would lose about 10 to 15 pounds through it all. It made it easy to keep a good figure. Those were the "bad old days."

I never heard the words "complex partial" until I was in my late 20s. The "white coats" (doctors) called my seizures "episodes," and some of them doubted they were even seizures. The first doctor I saw at age 13 told my parents there was nothing wrong with me, and I was probably on drugs. I was 17 when some doctors at a hospital threw water at me because I got upset and had a seizure. I was injected with the wrong medication at another hospital and then told I couldn't lie down.

If I had a seizure in public, I would always be brought to the hospital. I hated that. Their attitude was always that if you had a seizure, then it meant you either forgot to take your medication or that you were pregnant, drunk, or crazy. I laid on more gurneys explaining why I had a seizure and hoping the nurses (trained by the KGB) believed me. More than one doctor questioned why I didn't bite my tongue. It couldn't be a real seizure if I didn't bite my tongue, they announced. I had a CT scan once and got up from the table and fell on my face. The technician walked out of the room. I crawled out into the waiting room to my father and he picked me up off the floor. It seems I was allergic to the dye, something they only later discovered.

Then there was "the Loser." Some time ago, I met a man and we started seeing each other. I wasn't very interested in him, but it had been rather slow for me in the dating department. He was older than I was, balding, and not in the best of shape. But then again, I wasn't perfect either.

After we had been seeing each other around 3 weeks, I figured I had better tell him that I had seizures, because I would be having one pretty soon, and I would need to explain why I wouldn't be around for the next 5 or 6 days. At that time, I was having seizures once a month, and the entire episode would last for about a week.

I had always been told not to tell people about my seizures, but I felt it was only fair to let people know in case something happened. I had never had people react badly to it before, at least not to my face.

Well, he called me, and as we were talking, I told him I had epilepsy. He didn't even know what it was. I never met anyone who didn't know something about it. I explained what it was and what happened to me when I had seizures. I thought that was it.

We made a date to meet at a restaurant near his house that next Friday night. I sat at the table and went to order a drink from the waitress, and he stopped me. He told the waitress we changed our minds, and we weren't staying. Then he told me he couldn't deal with the fact that I had seizures and didn't want to see me anymore. He said it bothered him so much he had called "Ask-a-Nurse," and they had explained the condition to him.

All I felt was anger. This man that I didn't even want to date didn't want me because I have seizures. He can't hold a conversation, he is nothing to look at, he is no great charmer, and he acts like epilepsy is contagious. I got up from the table and walked out of the restaurant. I don't think I have ever been so insulted in my life.

"Loser" called me several times about a year after that to ask me out again. It seems he realized breaking up with someone because they have epilepsy or any other condition is pretty stupid. His loss.

It would surprise you to find out what bothers me when I have seizures. Not the more obvious things like "Will I die?" or "Will it hurt?" No, it's none of those. What has driven me crazy for years is having a feeling of knowing something occurred but not remembering it. I would have a week of seizures, after which I would know that an event occurred, but I could not remember the event happening. I know it sounds strange, but that is the only way I can describe it. This bothered me more than having a hundred seizures. I kept asking my doctor about it, whatever doctor I was seeing at the time. I usually got some lame "doctorese" speak about how my temporal lobe was in the cerebral cortex or something stupid like that. I came to the conclusion that either the doctors didn't know or didn't care, and I was going to have to figure it out myself.

I did, one night while watching the television show *M*A*S*H.* The plot line involved one of the characters having nightmares that turned out to be triggered by some moldy smelling uniforms. The episode got me thinking about college and the psychology class I had to take. Part of that class was about memory and what it is made up of. I had my answer: I was remembering the event, but it was just a memory I didn't recognize. During the times when I am in an active seizure, my senses do not function properly; they are either heightened or not working well at all. After the seizure is over, my senses return to normal. When I tried to recall a memory from a seizure, I couldn't, because my senses were so off during the seizure. It wasn't until the *M*A*S*H* episode that I was reminded that when you remember something, your mind must recall all of the senses in order to produce the memory.

I have too many horror stories to write about. Besides, it hurts to think about them. Of all the cruelties that epilepsy brings, most have nothing to do with the condition itself. The very people who are supposed to help are the ones who deliver most of the cruelties. I wish for two things: first, that all of these monsters get permanent yeast infections, and second, that God reserves a special place in Hell for them.

26

(Age 26) After being diagnosed with petit mal seizures at the age of 11, I grew up often wondering if I would have a normal adult life. Would this impair day-to-day routines such as learning, working, or driving, or my being able to have a family some day?

While in high school and college, I found that getting an education was serious and hard work. It was a chore that I despised, even today. It would take me three times longer than other people to study and achieve the grades that I wanted. Even though college was a challenge, I was able to graduate from a university. Now I'm a paramedic and love emergency medicine. Epilepsy has no effect on my professional life. The only problem I have from time to time is feeling fatigued from the medication.

Today I am 26 years old and married. Although we have no children, having epilepsy will not affect my family planning. I have a college degree and a professional job, love to ski down hill, and am able to drive a car. I am very fortunate that I'm able to live an independent and healthy life. Also, I'm able to have great relationships with my family and friends.

27

(Age 74) I am going to try to fill you in on my past long life regarding my seizure disorder.

When I was young, I just used to stare. Then I developed convulsions as I grew older. My mother always kept my problem a big secret from everyone. She was ashamed and so I felt the same way.

My seizures didn't affect dating or marriage because I always kept them in the closet. My husband and I were married 50 years ago. I never thought we would have children, but we had our first child 7 years later and our second child 4 years after that.

My disorder might have had something to do with my menstrual cycle, which was never normal or regular. One year, I went 9 or 10 months without having a period, and then I had a very heavy one for a couple of weeks. One summer, I had my period for about 2 months.

Years ago, I tried to overcome my feelings and went to work; I wouldn't pay attention to the way I was feeling. But now I put my feelings and myself first and my family accepts me. (I think!) Since learning more about epilepsy, I also don't mind telling people about it. Everyone seems to be sympathetic and understanding except one of my friends. Since I confided in her, she doesn't seem to want to be with me as much as she did before she knew. Her visits used to be daily, but now she comes by maybe once a month. This hurt me a great deal, but I am trying to rise above it.

I have been on my seizure medication for about 50 years. It has affected my balance and walking. A test confirmed that I had neuropathy as well as a back problem, for which I have had an operation.

I am 74 now and still trying to find a drug that will give me better control of my seizures. I know I am a burden to my family and this keeps them from going places, but they are the best!

28

(Age 38) Because of my epilepsy, my family felt an increased sense of obligation to me, to the point of suffocation. This has affected all aspects of my family life. Here are some examples of their interactions with me, which I acutely feel:

- They either denied my epilepsy or never talked about it— never ever talked about it.
- It caused a permanent anxiety to settle in that everyone struggled with. What should their part or role be? How should they change with the ups and downs—"ons and offs"—of this changing physical relationship? Therefore, in exasperation, people would distance themselves from me, or scold me for not having the same recognizance as the day before, that I was somehow doing "this" on purpose.
- Sometimes there was no support at all for me, for example, around issues like travel, exercise, work, or children.
- On the other hand, sometimes so much "support" was given to me that my interests were manipulated toward what was

thought to be "good for me." I was pushed toward an early marriage so my family could be secure in my care and accommodations, sort of like marrying off the eldest or ugliest daughter as a relief, saving the family from further embarrassment.

I have reacted in a couple of different ways. At times I behaved in an obedient, childlike mode because it was safe and nonconfrontational, or because I felt beaten. At other times I rebelled, knowing that taking any risk was completely my own responsibility and, at the very least, was causing dreadful anxious suffering for those around me (who would eventually have to aid me). This reaction had the potential for setting up a love/hate relationship.

Eventually, one way or another I would "give in" to others, definitely out of guilt. I never outgrew this from adolescence.

It seems that the nature of having epilepsy, like any special gift or disability, is upsetting to whole family systems due to ignorance about seizures and their treatment. It parallels the effects of alcoholism on a family. I know, because I married into that world and helped to sustain that whole sick, stunted way of life, for lack of knowing what else to do.

Friends have always come easy to me. Or at least acquaintances have. In general I like people and am fascinated by everyone. I don't spend time thinking about it, but I truly enjoy the odd person on the bus or old lady on an airplane who wants to chat. I like where people come from and what they have to say. Generally, I look for goodness in people and there is much of it to be found.

But when I get too close to people, things change. I try too hard and am too childishly eager for their approval; then I get embarrassed and am too open with them. Yet I think the positive side to having epilepsy is that perhaps it does increase your openness with others and a perceptibility, or sensitivity, toward people. Maybe this vulnerable openness attracts people because it is rarely critical or confrontational.

But then, usually around 6 months into a friendship, I begin to sense all the ignorance and tiresome misunderstandings that require endless explanations about why I fall down on my head. As people experience my epilepsy, they begin to see it's quite difficult to have a relationship with me. Usually the friendship dies. It's getting hard anymore to expect a lasting friendship, or to even try for it.

Here is the usual script.

1. I meet someone new who shares a common interest with me.
2. We go to a few events and my dependent, sad nature is revealed.
3. Usually there is a misunderstanding over some limitation of mine, like leaving early to go home and sleep or not committing to some activity.
4. They try to "fix me," not listening to me about what epilepsy is.
5. There is an argument and we go separate ways.
6. I am lonely.

I have very few friends. But there are people I consider my friends, and am confident they feel the same way about me. They

1. Have known me a long while and so have a "feel" for how I operate.
2. Don't expect apologies and are glad to see me. They let me be glad to see them each time we meet without judgment.
3. Allow me to call when I can continue the relationship (say it has been interrupted due to illness or a simple need like extra sleep).
4. Really do have an interest in how this "thing" epilepsy affects me; they listen to me and ask questions.
5. Allow me to ask about their lives, too.
6. Treat me no differently than any other friend.

I really don't understand sex. I thought I did. Certainly I understand the mechanics of it and the consequences of unsafe sex. But no one ever talked about "sex for the disabled," or the emotions generated thereof and how to sort this all out. Dare I suggest that the silence about it, coupled with abortion counseling in case I became pregnant, gave me the impression that sexual fulfillment for disabled people like me was sick and dirty?

After hearing a doctor speak, I began to move away from these ideas and look at my situation as it exists. This feels healthy. Perhaps sexuality for disabled people is not hopeless, and I am not alone in fear.

- I believe a disproportionate number of people with epilepsy are miscounseled, if at all, about reproduction.
- I believe some people vulnerable to seizures are easily manipulated and objects of sexual abuse.
- I believe women with epilepsy need the same accommodations during sex that are necessary with any other vigorous activity, such as time to be aroused and time to engage, as well as reassurance about the differences in orgasms that they may have. Women with epilepsy need to feel from their partner that it's all right to sexually respond as they are able.
- Partners should discuss the above so they can comfort each other, love each other over a long period of time despite changing events, and move from having children and parenting to menopause and golden old age.

Independence seems to be at the foundation of all the problems of people with epilepsy, or at least mine. Independence has been described as an inherently essential part of good communication, self-confidence, and decision making. It also has been the most elusive of qualities to attain for people with disabilities—and the first attacked by the public, so that we "stay under control" and "out of the way." Yes, there are the Americans with Disabilities Act (ADA) and civil rights, but favorable decisions based on these laws are only grudgingly awarded.

At first, lack of independence did not affect me. I did not associate it, or learn to associate it, with epilepsy. Consequently, I went right out into the world with whatever plans seemed appropriate for my age, like working throughout school, securing a driver's license, and hoping and dreaming like most people do. But things changed. The message to me was I ought not consider work or children or even worry about finishing school. I sought out counsel and went to the brightest people around me, who advised me to keep on trying. I should have considered it.

My reaction instead was to binge. I vehemently insisted on staying in school until I had a degree. I would spend as many weekends as I could pursuing entertainment that lasted all night or required me to drive 100 miles. I made sure I had a job and kept my own doctor's appointments. I grabbed at life. Now I know it would have been better to go slow, in increments, and gain self-reliance.

My ultimate goal was to have a family and to let people know no one was going to stop me. I could let go of graduate work, a career, and a car, but not the idea that I could not be married and have a family. I began dating, with the goal of having a baby. Epilepsy affected my normal dating development. I had extreme feelings of unworthiness and tremendous confusion over how to deal with what was happening to me and to "us" (and the whole concept of "us"). I also found it hard to explain epilepsy for an "us" situation.

I dated a lot of guys in sporadic relationships, and since I was bent on my own will, I didn't have long-term dating experiences. They lasted 3 or 4 months at most and then the "friendship pattern" of disintegration set in. I realized marriage would have to be swift. I still thought some miracle man would understand it all after dating me for a couple months. Not so.

I eventually did get married, but the marriage became impacted by the fact that we did not recognize the importance of communication. There were financial and spiritual casualties because of a complete misunderstanding of how to be married and be someone with epilepsy. I have learned that prior to a long-term commitment, all aspects of epilepsy must be discussed—treatment, payment plans, accommodations, and most importantly, the need for expressions of love. Maturity is necessary to balance any relationship. But an extra amount is needed when one person has a disability.

I always felt I could work to support myself. For me, epilepsy did not factor into whether or not I could work. Yet I never tried to support myself fully, completely independent of my family, as many people do in their 20s. I sought marriage not as a means of support, but as a route to familial happiness. So it was not until 15 years later (now) that I began searching for employment with realistic goals in mind such as providing for children or for retirement and receiving benefits.

I find the difficulty is not in becoming employed or going through the interview process, but rather in staying employed. I have had problems negotiating terms like pay and being mistaken as drunk or intoxicated (when in fact I was having seizures).

Accommodations in the workplace are different now than they were 20 years ago, but they still fall short for people with epilepsy. I look for organization, activities at a relaxed pace, few (if any) loud noises, nonblinking computer screens, proper (not glaring) lighting, and some way (like using a tape recorder) to review project plans as many times as I need to.

I believe, not think, that anything is possible.

29

(Age 50) "Ruth Ann, who's the President?"
"Uhhh, John Kennedy?"
"You think so? Who did you vote for?"
"Jimmy Carter?"

This exchange is the first memory I have after the automobile accident that began my journey into epilepsy.

It was 19 years ago. Doctors were asking the questions. At the time, I was terrified. They knew my name, but I did not recognize anyone. It seemed every answer I gave was wrong, and the doctors joked with each other, unaware that I thought they were causing the pain ripping through me. I thought if I remembered who the president was then they would stop hurting me.

To this day, I do not remember the accident. I'm thankful for that. Sometimes an incredible terror will swell up inside of me and I am afraid I *will* remember. I'd rather not.

I have no chronological memory of events over the next few years. Incidents come to mind haphazardly, and when I remember something, I ask my husband to explain it. He was in the accident also, and remembers everything...unfortunately.

When I regained awareness of my surroundings, which I am told was several days after the accident, I saw a man in the next bed. I was very agitated and annoyed. I tried to ignore him, but he insisted on talking. He said we were in the hospital. I told him he was a liar because they didn't put men and women in the same room in hospitals. He said it was okay because he was my husband. My husband?! Why didn't I remember him? He said we had three sons. Really, I thought. I did remember one child. I told him that if he was my husband, he would get out of bed and get us out of there. I did not understand that he was in traction with a broken hip. I lied to the doctors, and would have told them anything to get out of the hospital.

While in the hospital, I didn't always recognize family and friends. Folks have told me many stories of things I did and said that they were told to ignore because "I would be better soon." The problem was, I didn't get better soon.

For months, I would not allow friends into the house unless their name appeared on a list I carried around. Everything had to be written down: who was stopping by, where the children were, what I should and should not do.

The most vivid emotions I experienced were terror and confusion. I was so frightened I would hide in the closet. I could not understand what was real and what was imagined.

Until many months later, I had no emotional regard for anyone on a consistent basis. My husband's suffering was not a reality for me. Then, after a long time had gone by, I saw the scar on his hip. It was as if I was seeing it for the first time. When I asked how he got it, he was shocked. He had to explain his surgery to me, and then I cried. To think I had never offered him any love or comfort when it happened! I am astonished at how upsetting it is to think of this even now, so many years later.

When I think of the heartache I caused my husband, our sons, and our parents, it actually makes me physically ill. And it still makes me angry that the original doctors didn't help us. I went to one of them and told him I wasn't right. I attempted to explain the times I stared blankly, the way I seemed to fixate on a color, how motion made me cold inside. He said a near-death experience often made people question life and suggested we seek marriage counseling.

From what I know now, I must have been having seizures for some time. The little ones were not so noticeable, but they got progressively worse. Finally, my family physician saw me have one, and then prescribed phenobarbital. It was long after the accident, and when my mother saw the prescription, she said it was a tranquilizer given to neurotic people. So to her this meant that all I had to do was get my act together and I'd be fine. Of course, this made me feel worse.

I am thankful I was married and had children before I developed epilepsy. I can't imagine dating someone and having to tell him I might have a seizure. I probably would have become a nun. Fortunately, my husband is an extremely patient man. His patience and God's presence have preserved our marriage.

My life has two parts: one before the accident, and the other after the accident. Having seizures has changed me. What I was, I am not now.

Before, I was independent and confident. Now, I am dependent on my husband and others for transportation, which has a great impact on work-related issues. My confidence level has declined considerably because I fear having a seizure in front of people. I feel insecure and vulnerable.

Whenever I am going to be alone with my young grandsons, my sons will ask, "Have you taken your medicine?" Undoubtedly, their confidence in me has been shaken. No amount of assurance can erase the memory of the fall-down, out-of-control seizures they witnessed.

For 12 years, I worked as a preschool teacher. Having epilepsy affected many aspects of my work. Never was I allowed to be alone with the children. This affected my value as an employee; for example, I could not take my turn closing up. As owner and operator of a center, I had to pay someone to be with me regardless of whether or not I needed the help. Actually, I became ingenious at using extra help.

Perhaps the most disheartening incident occurred when two families saw me have a seizure. Soon after, they withdrew their children from the preschool, making feeble excuses for doing so. People are very squeamish about seizures. Having them tends to somehow lessen one's reliability and credibility in the view of others.

Over the years, we've begun to laugh more about the places I've had seizures and the peculiar ways people have reacted. Only in this last year have I begun to use the word "epileptic." Prior to seeing my current neurologist, I never used it and rarely ever told anyone I had seizures.

A new adventure for me now is menopause! How will I know if symptoms are due to seizure activity, side effects of medication, or hormonal changes? Thank God for good doctors, good friends, and a wonderful family.

30

(Age 48) Although my seizures are relatively mild and generally occur only once a week, they have significantly impacted several aspects of my life.

It is important to note that my seizures are a consequence of emergency brain surgery that was done to remove a tumor. Therefore, some of the emotional trauma associated with my seizures is hard to separate out from the medical emergency of the surgery itself and the fear that is still with my family and me. As one of my sons said, "Every time you have a seizure, it reminds us that you have brain cancer."

A large part of my work in the past involved counseling children at school. In fact, I was the supervisor of the counseling department before my diagnosis. The administration of the school decided it was best for me not to work alone with children out of concern that they would be upset or unsafe if I seized when I was with them. One child was, in fact, terrified by a seizure she observed.

I am no longer in the counseling department or working directly with children as I had done for the past 19 years. I have been given a different administrative position for which I have no specialized training. I am anxious about my ability to handle this work, because it requires good organizational skills and memory functions, two areas of deficit that I recently "acquired."

At home I have other concerns. I very much dislike my children being so concerned about me on a daily basis. Slight deviations in my body posture, movements, or affect may elicit the question, "Are you all right, Mom?" Once when I had closed my eyes to rest, it reminded one of my sons of the time I'd had my initial grand mal seizure and brought back unpleasant memories and feelings. On a recent vacation, my children worried about me having a seizure, even in the face of exciting and breathtaking scenery. My older son refused to go white-water rafting if I couldn't go, until I convinced him that this would make me feel worse. My husband, of course, also shares the stress that results from my seizures and has had to take on extra responsibilities as a parent, like driving.

When my seizures are more frequent, I often think "What will I do if I have a seizure now?" For example, I volunteer in my children's school as a presenter of a monthly program. I had to plan out carefully what to do if I began to have a seizure in front of my son's class. This, of course, increased my stress, and, consequently, my risk of seizing.

I will likely avoid these kinds of "public appearances" in the future. My friends and others outside my family seem to understand and accept my seizures, although they are certainly upset when they observe one. The seizures seem to happen when I am excited (for example, when I am out to dinner with friends). As a result, I wonder whether my son's playmates are less likely to be allowed by their parents to be under my care and supervision.

Being unable to drive has affected me greatly. I am dependent on others, especially my husband, to go almost anywhere (I live in the suburbs). My husband has become much more of a central parental figure because of this. Since he resents this, it has caused significant stress within our family. I find it very difficult to ask friends all the time because I do not want to strain our friendships. I use public

Personal Stories

transportation often and sometimes take expensive cab rides when all else fails.

Being sick and having cancer has changed me in many ways. I generally appreciate life and I love people much more. My "complaints" about seizures need to be seen in that context. If seizures are the price I pay for surviving brain cancer, I'm more than willing. My dependency on others—especially for driving—has been mostly infuriating, although I've also learned the extent of people's generosity and love for me; this has changed my understanding of human connectedness tremendously.

In this sense, ironically, my self-esteem has improved somewhat from having epilepsy because I feel more loved and like an important member of my community and extended family. Since I need to walk more, work less, and generally take better care of myself, I have had to learn to lead a healthier, slower paced, and more restful lifestyle, which I greatly enjoy.

Of course, the seizures themselves give me a terrible sense of loss of control. I feel terrible during and somewhat after. There is also a self-consciousness of how ugly they must make me seem and a sense of shame of having been seen this way. I think strangers must see me as defective. I worry that it affects the image that my family has of me in some subtle way.

I'm angry about the way the multiple medications make me feel. My changing neurological state, even during one day, disturbs me and takes up too much of my consciousness. Cognitive side effects of the medications cause me to feel (and be) less effective, and I've often made rather serious mistakes due to my faulty memory processing. My children are seeing me as less competent, and we all rely more on my husband. I resent this shift of power back to him.

I also have had to grieve for some things that I don't think I can do anymore, such as white-water rafting, climbing mountains, and riding a bike. I never know how cautious I need to be. I am hopeful that with better seizure control I will be less limited.

I appreciate the love of my family more than ever, but I do feel less of a person than before. I can sum this up with something my younger son said to me recently: "You're not as much fun as you used to be, Mommy, but I still love you."

31

(Age 44) Growing up, I had a hard time in school with the other students and trouble making friends because they were afraid of getting near me. They thought they could "catch" epilepsy.

Now that I have children, I find that explaining all about my seizures to them and repeatedly saying that I'll be fine if I have a seizure makes it easier for them to accept my epilepsy.

My seizures are usually followed by a deep sleep for 3 hours. Just before my menstrual cycle, I usually have a few more seizures than usual, which I think is due to more fluids in my body.

32

(Age 19) Here are the burning questions about my epilepsy that I have struggled with throughout my life:

- Why do I have to take so many pills?
- Why do I still have seizures after taking all the medication?
- Will I be able to have children?

It is very hard to me to face the reality that I am 19 years old and yet do not have the right to drive. Whenever I watch my 16-year-old brother drive, I think to myself, "It's just not fair!" I think that's the hardest thing for me to deal with.

Having seizures scares me, but dealing with my lack of driving makes me depressed. When I look at all the people on the road driving their own cars, like my friends, I feel different.

33

(Age 47) I have had seizures for the past 21 years, and I'm sure that this has had a big impact on my life. I'm always afraid that I'll have a grand mal, even though I have only had one (about 17 years ago, when my youngest son was born).

I've always kept most of this information about myself private. I didn't want anyone else to know this about me, since I thought they'd think "less" of me. When I went to see the local neurologist, I'd pray I wouldn't meet anyone I knew, because then I'd have to explain where I was going and why.

Even my husband didn't understand—he either thought it was a joke or wouldn't talk about it at all, thus encouraging me not to talk about it and be ashamed. My mom wouldn't talk that much about it, calling it a "spell."

Today I still have terrible feelings about my having seizures because of this lack of full understanding from my family. Even so, I think I'm becoming more accepting of my diagnosis; I recently shared with a friend of mine some of my feelings about my diagnosis of "epilepsy." It's probably because I am starting to feel better about myself.

I know that even though I have epilepsy, or the more preferable term, "seizure disorder," I am still a worthwhile person.

34

(Age 61) Epilepsy was like a veil through which I saw myself, life, and even the God for whom I sought to live. People who loved me always surrounded me, but I felt less than acceptable, unable to truly appreciate their love, and certainly unable to fathom why I was loved. For years I had felt that seizures put up the barriers of fear and shame. I recognized, finally, that something within me was a blockage to inner peace, and sought help in therapy.

I was 9 years old at the time of my first seizure. For the next 10 years, I had petit mals ten or more times a day and grand mals several times a year. Today I am 61 years old. My seizures are well controlled by medication and by trying to avoid the stresses that trigger them.

When I was in my 30s, I heard it said that the greatest development in the field of epilepsy was physicians' "awareness" of the psychosocial aspects of epilepsy. Immediately, I realized that if physicians lacked this awareness in the past, then no wonder there was no one to help my parents cope with my epilepsy! I also sensed immediately that the lack of this insight had left a major mark on my life. That comment helped me understand my parents' dilemma, but it was 20 more years before I really confronted my own.

It was a painful process, but in the end it was a great relief. I burdened myself with too much unnecessary guilt. It's good to realize there are some things I cannot change, and good to have help trying to change others.

In the 1940s and 1950s, troublesome feelings and issues were not talked about openly. There was no understanding of the side effects of medication. My mother was terribly afraid for me; I sensed it and tried to hide my fear from her. I was successful at this, because she never knew. (I asked her when I was about 58). To this day, I *still* hide any seizure activity from her.

She carried the burden as her own for most of her life. My brother was never told I had epilepsy until I mentioned it in adulthood. His wife told me he'd spent his childhood wondering what was wrong with his sister and wanting to help. Today I feel we *all* suffered because of unexpressed grief. It seems to me that epilepsy is an "-ism" in the family and all are affected, much like the "-ism" of alcoholism. Both involve enormous control. I grew up appearing to be very "strong-willed" but feeling enormously dependent. I did seek and find lifelong closeness to other extended family members. I wonder: Did waiting for the next seizure make my whole family "uptight?"

At a very early age, years before I began having seizures, I had a great desire in my heart to be "very close to God." I had strong influences in my family in this regard. Perhaps the isolation I experienced from having epilepsy—and my enormous need for acceptance—intensified this longing. It became and has been the central part of my life. God, as I understand God, has led me to realize I was running from the sacredness of my humanity, and that feelings are a tool of the soul. I am convinced that I thought my feelings caused seizures, and so I tried to suppress them.

I've always had many friends, but found close personal relationships fraught with intense emotion, and tried to escape from them. After dating one young man (who is still a friend 40 years later), I found my way into a religious community of women who had various handicaps. Petit mals ceased very soon. I think freedom from stress and a deep sense of belonging helped. Then conflict came, and I left the community. I never grieved for that loss, either, until I learned to grieve during therapy.

I have lived alone for 27 years, finding fulfillment in belonging to groups, as well as in close friendships with women, avoidance of sexual interaction, and my work. Professionally, I have been very fortunate. When nursing was closed off to me because of seizures, I found medical technology to be a way for me to help in the care of the sick. Opportunities for ministry to the suffering and dying presented themselves to me all along the way; I feel my own inner suffering sensitized me to that of others. When I was in the community, I had great responsibilities, like running the lab single-handedly. But when I left, I actually hid my expertise, running from supervisory positions, desiring only to be a "team member." I have done that well, but now recognize that I do not have much energy left for life beyond work.

I do not cope well with the stresses of life, like the loss of my parents. My home is disorganized; I am often overwhelmed by the multitude of chores, and it's difficult to decide which ones to do first.

I persevered in therapy because I sought truth, and the most difficult truth for me to accept was the professional perspective that I have been depressed all my life, I just didn't know it (and neither did others). I was always seen as a very happy, peaceful person. Now I understand that dysthymia, a mild-to-moderate chronic form of depression, is part of my seizure disorder.

Someone once said, "How can you separate a yolk from the egg?" As I enter the last phase of my life, I am trying to decide what to do about this now, and I feel the pace of my work is too much for me. Therapy has taught me that change is a good thing, and part of life and growth.

With all my heart I applaud the Epilepsy Foundation, physicians, and all health care workers for their efforts to help parents and children address these issues and learn to deal with losses in their early years.

Personal Stories

Thank you for giving me the opportunity to write about epilepsy. It was a powerful experience for me to try to be concise in expressing some of the most important things in my life. I hope it will be helpful to you.

35

(Age 39) My diagnosis of epilepsy has affected my life in many different ways. When I have a seizure, I am usually not aware of what is happening. I become very disoriented, confused, and sometimes lost. I may black out and fall. Seizures are very unpredictable, and that makes them scary.

One morning I was standing on a bus. Before I realized it, I was in an ambulance. Apparently, I had a seizure on the bus, which was frightening to me. As usual, I had no forewarning (aura) that would have let me known the seizure was coming.

It is very difficult to have epilepsy. It has affected my social life by putting up a shield between my friends and myself. And I feel that I am putting a huge weight on their shoulders because I have epilepsy. When I address the problem, I feel very nervous and embarrassed because I don't know how to even deal with my feelings about my seizures. The fact that they are very unpredictable makes me pull away from people more. I do not want to scare people; rather, I want them to feel comfortable around me. That's why I want the seizures to be under control before I have any close relationships.

It is disconcerting to me that I have no auras. Seizures hit me like lightning. I could be doing something very important, and then all of a sudden a seizure takes place. I am aware of what can contribute to triggering my seizures, such as stress, caffeine, fever, and missing a dose of medicine.

I am also very angry that my life is limited due to my seizures. When I was in my 20s, I wanted to join the Peace Corps after I got my teacher's degree. I wanted to teach the children and learn about their culture. I never got to undertake that challenge. There have been other situations where the seizures stood in the way of a challenge, like traveling abroad to see friends. I am going to work hard so I can make these challenges a reality.

The most difficult thing about having seizures is living in fear of them. I wonder every day whether or not it will be a calm day, neurologically. When I wake up and start to travel in the morning, I become concerned about the possibility of a seizure suddenly happening. It is very difficult to deal with the fear. I wish I had auras so I could prepare for the seizures. I also wish that the seizures were better controlled, but this is what is being worked on.

Hopefully, I won't have to live in a dark tunnel much longer and the light will shine for me much brighter one day.

36

(Age 41) I am very blessed to have God in my life, first of all, and a wonderful spouse. My family relationships have not been affected by epilepsy.

The last time that I had a major episode with epilepsy was 20 years ago. My husband never even knew that I had epilepsy. I kept it from him until the seizures happened. I was taken to the hospital, and that is where my husband found out. He was surprised—but also wonderful—about it and did not allow it to affect our marriage.

Of course, we then spoke about my seizures, but he explained to me that I should not have kept something like this a secret from him because I could not help being sick.

At the time my husband found out about my seizures, I was 9 months pregnant with my son, who is now 21 years old. I had stopped taking the seizure medication a few months before, and I believed that is why I had the seizures. The doctors told me to start taking the medication again. I had stopped because I thought that it would affect the baby. Eight years later I got pregnant again with my daughter. I was told not to stop the medication, and, thank God, my baby was not affected by the medication.

I don't let most people know that I have epilepsy. Those who do know do not really care. It doesn't affect our friendships.

I have not had any trouble getting jobs. I am independent because I have a spouse who pushed me into being independent. I do have some fears. I was afraid to drive, and now that I can, I will still not travel on highways.

I am learning every day to be more independent.

37

(Age 27) Devastation was the first thought that came into my mind when I became cognizant after my first grand mal seizure. Then came disbelief. I was 26 years of age and—I thought—healthy. Because I worked in the health care field, I had heard of epilepsy and seizures and knew it was not a good thing, but I had little understanding of it. Up until this seizure, there was no need. Nobody close to me was affected by it.

As I went through the tests, I thought everything was going to be all right, that what happened was not true. To hear the word *epilepsy* shook me to the core. This was unbelievable, so I got a second opinion: same diagnosis.

Epilepsy meant daily medications, blood checks, and no driving. I felt that my independence was gone. The lifestyle that once was mine was altered. Everything I did or wanted to do took thinking about; how I was going to get there, and how was I going to get home? These thoughts made me very discouraged and at times withdrawn. My family or friends had to be around to pick me up and drive me places. I felt like their lives were being affected by my problem. Public transportation took its toll on me. Running to catch a bus or a train, making connections with another, and finally walking to work wore me out. Nearly every day, the pace I had to keep agitated me.

At times when I felt good or "normal," I would worry deep down, "Am I really all right? Is the medication really working? Am I being monitored as best as I can be? Am I remembering to take my pills?"

Today, I am a little more confident and I don't have to whisper the word *epilepsy* when someone asks, as if it were a dark, terrible problem. I feel well supported by my neurologist, nurse, social worker, family, friends, and coworkers.

I am a single 27-year-old woman now. I am proud that I have coped with all the trials and tribulations of being diagnosed with epilepsy and monitored for over a year now. I wonder what my future holds—maybe career changes, relationships/marriage, family/children—and how my epilepsy will affect or not affect these life events, the people I will be meeting, and my future family members.

I am up-front about my diagnosis and express that I do not see it as a problem. I am on medication, well monitored, and supported. That, in itself, is reassuring to me as well as to others. I do not know what problems the future may hold, but now is not the time to

Personal Stories

worry about those things. I will cross those bridges when I come to them. I know that I have resources at my fingertips and a knowledgeable and well-rounded team of caregivers. I am more confident about my health than I was initially, and I don't feel set back at all. I have many to thank for that.

When I look ahead to the future, it is not grim because of epilepsy. It is bright as it was before my first seizure.

38

(Age 50) Epilepsy has had a major effect on me, from dating and romantic relationships, to marriage, menstrual function, pregnancy, family life, and friendships.

When I dated, I would not let on about my having epilepsy for fear of being rejected by the other person. If we continued dating, and he somehow found out about my epilepsy, I would explain to him what would happen to me if a seizure came on and what he would have to do. I would also reassure him so that he wouldn't be scared. I would tell him that my seizures aren't that bad and last only up to a minute and a half; after, I would come out of it and be confused for a while.

I was 17 years old when I started menstruating. My neurologist said it could have come late due to the medications I was taking. I felt so relieved to get it because I already felt different from my friends for having epilepsy; getting my period, even if it was late, at least made me more like my friends.

Over time, my cycle became regular and I realized that each month I would *always* have a few seizures 1 week before my period. These seizures, I felt, were a part of my menstrual cycle. They just automatically came the week before the menses each and every month. If my period was thrown off for some reason, so were these seizures. The seizures were like my premenstrual syndrome.

My husband and I always got along very well and were the best of friends before we got married. We didn't see eye to eye on everything, but always came to an agreement and seldom argued.

However, there was one important thing lacking in our marriage that I just couldn't do anything about: I had no desire for sex. I think it was due to the medications that I was taking for epilepsy. Only once in a great while, maybe four to five times a year, would I care for sex. I know this was so unfair to my husband, yet I couldn't change this or do anything about it. I'd have a hard time showing my feelings sexually, except for those few times each year that I could let go and show my feelings. At those times, I almost felt as though I was a nymphomaniac because I would enjoy it so much and would want it constantly! My husband could never understand this one thing about me, nor could I ever understand it myself. Now that they have Viagra for men, maybe something can eventually be discovered for my kind of problem.

Luckily, my ability to have children was not affected by my epilepsy. When I was pregnant with my first child (son), I didn't have any seizures for the whole 9 months that I carried him. That was the longest I had gone without a seizure since they started at the age of 12 years. When my son was born, he was in perfect condition, but he did have to take phenobarbital for a while because he was withdrawing from it. When I was pregnant with my second child (daughter), I had only a few seizures the whole 9 months of pregnancy. I was on different medications when I carried her, and she didn't have to be given anything when she was born.

Both pregnancies were easy for me, and I felt good during each of them—no morning sickness or anything like that. When my babies were infants, I was very nervous. If my husband was at home, he would carry them for me because I was afraid of a seizure while holding the baby. My husband, sisters, and friends would help me out a lot when our children were babies. I would carry them as little as possible because of that fear of dropping one. I felt a lot better when they learned to walk because of that fear.

My husband passed on 7 years ago due to alcoholism. My son Bill is now 22; my daughter Cheryl is 17. Both my children have quit school. Neither would listen to me, so they have to find out for themselves the hard way. My daughter plans to get her high school equivalency diploma when she is 18. At this time, she is working at a supermarket and my son at a produce store. My daughter has a nice boyfriend who she really likes and who is good to her. I don't worry too much about her like I do Bill. I'm always worried about my son because of drug and alcohol problems. Also, I can see he is not a happy person. I've tried getting him to go to therapy, but he refuses to cooperate. I know for myself I need to go to Al-Anon. I have a problem with tough love, which everyone tells me my son needs. But that is hard for me. As a family, we don't do much together. We all seem to go our own way. When Cheryl's not at work, she is out with her boyfriend. When Bill's not at work, he's out with his friends.

My pastime is playing Keno with my sister Rose. We both enjoy gambling (too much!) but have to limit ourselves.

I had a partial hysterectomy last year. I'm going through "the change" now. I've only had hot flashes a couple of times. Some days I feel my age and some days I don't. My seizures haven't changed in any way.

Most of my family and friends are very understanding about epilepsy. But I do have a couple of relatives (an aunt and cousin) who are very ignorant when it comes to epilepsy. They think it is "all up to myself" or that it is "mind over matter" as to whether or not I have a seizure, and that I can control the seizures myself. At one time, I used to get angry and upset with them about this, but now I realize that they just don't understand the problem. In a way, I feel sorry for them.

When my husband was alive, he would drive me to my appointments or wherever else I needed to go, since I don't have a license to drive. Now, I've gotten used to public transportation and don't mind it at all. That was one way I depended on my husband, but otherwise, I've always been a very independent person. My epilepsy has never affected my being independent.

Living on a disability check can be hard and very frustrating. I feel as though I live from month to month, check to check. It's really hard some months to manage my money, because I never know what's going to come up that throws off my budgeting. It's a lot better to be able to work for your money and receive a check once a week.

I don't know if how I sometimes feel about myself has contributed to my epilepsy or not. I've always had low self-esteem and at times don't like myself. I can't look at anyone. I am paranoid at times when in public places. This has gotten worse as I've grown older. At times, I'm full of fear with a lot of anxiety; sometimes I know why I have it, but sometimes I don't.

When I was younger, my seizures made me feel that I was not as good as my siblings. We didn't get along sometimes, so they would joke about my epilepsy. Today we all laugh about it, and the names we had for each of us. But as a kid, I felt that they were all better than me.

What bothers me about a seizure is I'm always afraid that if I have one in a public place that I'll become incontinent with my urine. Once a seizure is over, it's over, but that problem is there and is very embarrassing. It really upsets me.

Besides affecting my sex drive, I think medications have affected my memory. My kids and husband would often tell me something, and I would forget. My husband would tell me about a meeting at work, and that he'd be late, and I'd forget. I would have to write a lot of things down.

Besides a pill for a low sex drive, I could sure use one for bad memory.

39

(Age 34) In many ways, I feel emotionally like a 16-year-old. I suppose it's understandable. I started having complex partial seizures when I was 3 years old. No doctor figured out I was having seizures until I was 21. I missed out on the opportunity to fully develop socially and emotionally during those years that I was living without any treatment for my undiagnosed seizures.

As a child, and particularly as a teenager, I was often described as "inattentive," "flippant," "disaffected," "underachieving," and "antisocial." I only later found out that all of those terms could be used to describe what happens to someone when they have complex partial seizures. The neurologist prescribed medication and sent me on my way. I was relieved to know that I wasn't crazy, and that many of my behaviors were not my fault and not within my control.

This was all well and good, but no seizure medication would bestow upon me social graces. The damage was done. I couldn't turn back the clock to the eighth grade to learn to flirt, or to the tenth grade to learn to date. All of these things are part of the necessary framework for forming meaningful relationships.

I was still having eight to ten complex partial seizures per day and missing many of the subtle social cues kids learn. When I was about 15, I was so frustrated that I tried to "self-medicate" with illegal drugs. I would also skip school in order to avoid the social agony of having so many complex partial seizures every day.

As a young adult, I couldn't hold down a job. I had a hard time maintaining a basic college course load and depended on my parents for everything. Worst of all, I was already on a downward spiral of relationships with men who were either married, physically abusive, substance abusers, or all of the above. Unfortunately, this trend continued well into my 20s. I was still having many seizures a day.

When I was about 26, I woke up one day—literally—and announced to my family that I was sick of living on social security disability, sick of doing nothing, sick of being isolated, and most of all, sick of being sick. If I was going to sit isolated at home and have seizures, then I could become a member of society and have seizures just as easily. I became determined to function in this world.

I decided to attend a 2-year college to learn architectural drafting, a field in great demand. I graduated and began my career as a computer-aided drafter. Although I was now able to hold down a meaningful job and earn a decent living, I was still making poor choices in relationships.

About 2 years ago, I dedicated myself to ending the poor choices in men that I was making. I haven't had a sexual relationship in 2 years. What I do have are friends—real friends—I can call and talk to. I have become more independent and confident. I live on my own—I have an apartment and a car. I've had the same job for 5 years.

Recently, I have been receiving an experimental drug. My seizures are finally coming under control. This has been a total eye-opener. I can't believe how much better I feel. It also feels good not having to make excuses for memory lapses and odd behaviors. When I meet new people, I'm not living in fear of embarrassing myself.

I even have a friend who is male and available. I feel like I'm 16 and learning to date. Only this time around, I'm seeing the social cues I was missing as a teenager.

I wouldn't trade what I'm feeling now for anything!

40

(Age 52) How have seizures affected my day-to-day life over the past 30 years? First of all, I was unable to function as a mother when my children were born because my seizures got worse and all I

Personal Stories

wanted to do was sleep. My sister-in-law and husband did everything for me. When the children started needing rides everywhere, I always had to ask other people, and I was stuck in the house and lonely.

Seizures affected our finances. I can't work a good paying job since I can't remember anything. Because of all the medication I take, I only have the energy to work 15 hours a week because it is tiring work, packing bags in a supermarket. I feel like a real loser because I can't make $30,000 a year like everyone else's wives. I can only make $3,000. When we are out with other people, I can't participate in any discussions because they are always talking about computers and topics of which I have no knowledge.

Seizures have affected my independence because I can't drive. I use the bus service now, but I don't want to go off alone somewhere in case I have a seizure. I am also unable to function as a wife for my husband because I'm just plain numb when it comes to sexual relations.

Finally, I only have three good friends because it is difficult to form relationships with people when they discover my medical condition.

And yet, I *can* enjoy life. I just got back from touring the Rockies on our motorcycle for the fourth time. It's so beautiful.

41

(Age 33) I have had epilepsy since I was 11 months old. When I began puberty, the seizures became less well controlled.

As a woman, I have found that seizures affect my menstrual cycle and my relationships. It has caused my menstrual cycles to be irregular and my seizures to increase the week before and the week of the cycle. In doing so, it causes my life to be interrupted both at work and at home. I take extra medication if this happens while I'm at work, but the added medicine and seizures will often cause me to change my sleeping habits. For example, to get the rest that I require, I'll need to take naps during the day and go to bed early.

The seizures affect my husband and my mother. My mother is always nervous when I am having problems and comes across doubting what I am capable of doing, which puts a strain on our relationship. Since my medication has not been able to get my seizures under control, my doctor put me on a study medication. As a result, I am not allowed to get pregnant or I will be taken off my new pills. This was an important decision that my husband and I had to make. We decided that it was more important to raise children than to become pregnant and have our own. So we decided to adopt a child.

To prepare to be a mother I had to take into account that my seizures may get in the way. As a result, we needed to organize our home so that each area of our house had a safe area to put a child. I generally get a warning prior to my seizure, and it is during this time that I would place a child in a safe area. This means having a playpen on the first floor and a crib and bassinet upstairs, one in each room. It also means organizing the infant's care with my husband, so he will be responsible for bathing our child in the tub when I am having difficulties.

Both my seizures and medications have caused me to experience mood swings. This happens when I have been having a lot of seizures. I become upset and often depressed. This makes me change my daily routine, including any special activities that my husband and I had planned for each other.

I have taken medication that has caused me to sleep more and others that have given me insomnia. In each case, my husband and I had to change our evening routine. When I had insomnia, I took up sleeping in our guest bedroom so I wouldn't keep him up. When

I required more sleep, I ended up going to sleep before he did, so we wouldn't see a lot of each other in the evening.

As a woman, I have also experienced a lowering of my sexual drive and need. I have been fortunate enough to have a loving husband who doesn't put a lot of stress or demand on me in this area and accepts me the way I am. We had explored this topic when we first got married. It has been explained to me that this could be a result of my epilepsy and/or medications. This has always been part of me and I have had to accept it.

42

(Age 47) Discovering that I had epilepsy affected my life in many ways, on many levels. The first shock of it had its impact on my self-esteem and self-image. So little appeared to be known about temporal lobe epilepsy at that time, and what was known was profoundly negative. One medical research book I consulted claimed that it led to retardation. Adding to that, my mother (born in 1913) forbade me from telling anyone in the family about my illness; so shame was blended with fear.

Naturally, all of this eventually affected my relationships. My husband of only 2 years found his fidelity to the vow of "in sickness and in health" wavering when he heard the diagnosis. He tried to convince me that I was just "nervous." My marriage was on thin ice, anyhow, and epilepsy added the final crack. We separated a year and a half later.

From that point on, staying employed and independent were my top priorities; relationships were the furthest thing from my mind.

I tried many different medications. Their terrible side effects made me constantly afraid of losing my job, and because I had no support system and no family to speak of, it was even more frightening. Much of the time, I had employers who were understanding, but sometimes there was bias against me because of the condition. Resumes were handed back to me when I said the ugly "E" word, and once I lost a job after 3 weeks, with no notice, when my memory skills were found to be deficient. So I have always had great anxiety about money.

As I move toward the age of 50, the relationship matter becomes more important. However, I have very little hope I will ever find a partner. Being 47 makes it hard enough, but having epilepsy on top of my age renders the situation nearly hopeless.

Epilepsy makes one "unmarketable," both for jobs and emotional sustenance. It is a very lonely illness. I am resigned to the loneliness, but the resulting financial insecurity is harder to live with. Looking ahead to the not-so-distant future when I can no longer work is horrifying. With no savings, retirement plan, or helpful family members, I will surely end up in some state-assisted facility—a very grim prognosis.

Medications and treatment have improved tremendously since I developed epilepsy, but the impact of epilepsy on one's personal life is still so hard. When you don't know from one moment to the next if you are going to be fully conscious for the next 5 minutes, you become very anxious and jumpy. Relaxation techniques are helpful, but ultimately it is out of one's control—the brain cells do whatever they damn well please.

So my life as a woman with epilepsy is uncertain, lonely, and scary. Good thing the condition has left me devoid of any desire for sex. Otherwise, I'd be much lonelier.

43

(Age 36) My grand mal seizures started when I was 15. Looking back, that was probably the worst age for me to begin having seizures. High school can be a scary place—even without epilepsy—and I was shy to begin with. I withdrew further into myself, never once dating. I was terrified that a seizure would happen in school, or that someone would discover my terrible secret. Luckily, that didn't happen. Still, I missed proms and all the other exciting events that go with being a teenager.

In my 20s, I started dating. One relationship became serious, and I became concerned about having a seizure in front of my unsuspecting boyfriend. I was also unsure how to tell a potential husband that I could not have children, since I was too scared of the effect my medication would have on the baby.

I attempted to broach the subject, but before I could get anywhere, my boyfriend, put off by my tears, told me he didn't want to know. Later I met another man (now my husband) and received the concern and sympathy I desperately needed. I remember praying to God to keep me from having a seizure on my wedding day. He did.

At the age of 34, I became pregnant and worried myself through 9 months. My medication is known to increase the risks of birth defects in babies. More important, said my doctor, was to prevent a seizure while pregnant. There is no way to properly express how thankful I am for my two beautiful, healthy boys, born only 13 months apart.

Unfortunately, the two pregnancies took their toll, and in January of this year my seizures returned with a vengeance. Because of that, I now have someone with me at all times for my babies' safety. I am never alone with them and often don't feel I am a "complete" mother. My house is not my own. I can't drive while my seizures are active, so we are limited mainly to home activities.

Rest for me is extremely important, so my children never see my face in the middle of the night. The most common emotion I feel right now is guilt. I feel guilt that my husband is exhausted. I feel guilt that my mother and father drive 45 minutes each way three times a week to help me with the kids. I feel guilt that my kids are not out exploring the world with me.

But it is the not knowing when a seizure might occur that worries me daily. "Waking up" from a seizure is the most devastating feeling. I have no warning of my seizures, so waking up is the realization for me that I had a seizure, and I feel deeply depressed. Surely the phrase "pick yourself up and dust yourself off" should be the motto of someone with epilepsy. But I have learned over the years not to try to fight the sadness that comes after a seizure. It's part of a process that gets me going again.

Unfortunately, my memory seems to worsen after each seizure and I lose recall of certain things. Last year, I lost all memory for the several weeks that preceded a cluster of seizures, including memories of Christmas day. I look at other women and envy their properly functioning brains.

All that I've written sounds self-pitying, but it is the effect my seizures have had on me as a woman. A woman should be feminine and pretty. Seizures are ugly. Two of my friends who witnessed a seizure said it was the scariest moment of their lives. That's not an easy burden for me to carry.

Seizures have given me some things. I've become stronger emotionally. I know how truly lucky I am to have a wonderful, fun, supportive family. I have my beautiful, healthy boys and hope— hope that my doctor and I will find the right treatment to keep my seizures away. I recognize how things could be so much worse and that so many other people suffer from horrible, painful illnesses.

Personal Stories

44

(Age 44) When I first sat down to write this, I believed I had nothing to contribute. I have always tried to live my life as though epilepsy wasn't part of the equation. But I found myself saying "except for" a lot.

I see epilepsy from two perspectives. My cousin, Mary Anne, had a very severe case, worse than me. I hate to admit that before my own epilepsy surfaced, I would see my cousin go into seizures and I looked upon her with pity and some indifference, believing that somehow she had caused this to happen, and after all, God punished the evil. Although I believed she had been punished enough, she died of an attack at the age of 33, after falling into a bathtub full of water.

The other perspective is my own. I developed epilepsy at the age of 12. I believed that my epilepsy was different than my cousin's, and I spent my entire life trying to prove that I was normal, capable, intelligent, and loving.

Given how I felt about watching my cousin have seizures, what I feared most was that the impact of watching me have a seizure would be too much to bear for friends, family, and strangers. I always tried to jump up after a seizure in the hope of making others believe that I was OK and not different. I wanted the seizure to be looked at as if I had just fainted from the "vapors," rather than a person thrashing on the floor with a contorted face.

I didn't like telling other parents that I had epilepsy, because usually that meant their kids were always somewhere else when I came around to play. I just tried to forget that I was epileptic. Even at a young age, I realized it was better to keep my mouth shut and hope I was lucky enough not to have a seizure.

My parents and siblings were great in that they never treated me different unless I went into a seizure. Then, they would all cry. I would wake up, surrounded on all sides of the bed by my family. I am very lucky like that. I depended on my family to be "my life" because I got acceptance. However, I always believed that underneath, they hoped I would marry someone who would accept me and take care of me.

This made me want to prove that I could do anything. I taught myself how to type and then went to secretarial school (and then on to medical transcription, which wasn't my thing, although I was very good at transcription).

I did finally marry a man. I will always love him to my last breath—my husband Albert. We were married exactly 3 months and 9 days when he took his own life and jumped off a bridge. I had fought depression my whole life, but this was a defining moment for me. I couldn't keep him alive.

Sometime after that, I tried to be better, happier, and healthier, at least for those around me. My husband's suicide only reconfirmed that the outside world didn't want me. I had to change. During my search for improvement, I read a medical book on epilepsy that said up until the late 1960s, people with epilepsy could not legally be married. They were considered mentally defective.

I was more determined then ever to be the best I could be, at least on the outside. So I was the person that everyone came to when something went wrong in the family. I took people in when things went wrong. I tried to be there for my family in every way. Right after my husband's death, I went to live with my aunt who was dying of cancer. Her own kids couldn't even deal with it.

I married again, and with some encouragement from Philip, I started trying to improve myself again. He was fairly intelligent, so I wanted to get a college education that would make me "equal to him" intellectually. I got my degree in accounting and in my first year of college, he left me for my "best friend." Maybe I would feel I was worth something, if only people stopped leaving me for one reason or another.

I was determined to make the "outside" world my foe, or at best a distant stranger, never to be let into my life again. I stopped fighting the negativity and took it in until it became my life. Maybe it was a matter of bad judgment, but a combination of epilepsy, public perception, depression, and a lack of self-esteem has brought me to this point.

Now it is just a matter of buying time.

45

(Age 32) I started having seizures when I was 24 years old. I had just returned home from work and the phone rang. It was my friend, Denise. She asked me how I was feeling. I said, "Fine. Why?" Then she dropped a bomb on me. She asked, "Are you on drugs?" I said, "No! What are you talking about?" She explained, "You were acting very strange today at work when I was talking to you. You didn't hear a word I said—you just kept staring for about 7 minutes."

I started to cry and called my parents to tell them what happened. They took me to the hospital, where I had all kinds of tests. I was told that I had a seizure. I started crying again, because all kinds of things were running through my head.

I left the room to calm down and then went back into the doctor's office. I told him that I had a brain tumor removed when I was 4 years old, followed by radiation therapy. Growing up, I was fine and doing well in my classes. The doctor then said he would like to do an EEG on me.

After I had the EEG, my doctor told me that I probably had scar tissue on my left temporal lobe. He said that my birth control pills had triggered my seizures, so I stopped taking my birth control pills, hoping that the seizures would stop. But they didn't.

I saw the doctor again. I told him I was getting married in 2 more months. Could I be having seizures from all the excitement? He said it was possible. I hoped that after I got married, my seizures would stop because a lot of pressure would be gone. Well, they didn't stop—they just seemed to increase! My seizures didn't affect my relationship with my husband in any way. We kept a normal relationship. Some days I would get a little upset if my husband was at work or none of my friends or family were around, because I wouldn't go out by myself. I was afraid of having a seizure while I was crossing the street, or getting confused and lost.

Despite having seizures, I kept working at a bank in the payroll department. My seizures did not seem to affect my job. If I had a seizure at work, I would stop working and stare until the seizure stopped, and then I would continue where I left off.

The hardest thing for me was being unable to drive. I had to depend upon other people to get back and forth to work. I wouldn't go any place alone. One of the most important things I realized was who my real friends were, because I lost some so-called friends when I started having seizures.

I also noticed that my personality had changed. I was very moody. The scary thing for me was that I felt like I didn't know myself. I had no idea when a seizure was about to come on. If I was alone, I wouldn't know whether I had had one or not.

A couple of years ago, I went to see my neurologist. I told him that I wanted to start a family. I had about a hundred questions to ask him. The most important one was whether my seizures were hereditary. He said no. Then I asked if the medication I was taking could affect my baby, and he said it was very unlikely.

Personal Stories

Well, during my pregnancy, I had no seizures and no problems. We had a beautiful baby boy. He is a very special baby in our life, and he is as healthy as can be. I love being a mother and seeing that my epilepsy hasn't affected my son in any way.

It has now been 5 years since I had a seizure!

46

(Age 49) Epilepsy is so new to me that I don't know what experiences merit sharing. At this time, there has been relatively minimal effect on the quality and substance of my life. Until this point, I've been fortunate to be in good health and not to take medication beyond an aspirin or acetaminophen here and there. It took a while to get adjusted to taking medication on a schedule and remembering to take it with me at the start of the day.

I lead a busy life with a hectic work and personal schedule. Life continues as before I had epilepsy. I work as an independent consultant and keep the same hours and continue to travel, just as before. My relationship with my husband has not changed, nor has my life with our two sons, with one exception: I seem to be more sensitive to the heat, and this has limited my playing baseball with our younger son. Then again, it's been a particularly hot few weeks, so this may just be a function of heat mixing with age.

The initial seizures occurred when I was visiting my parents. Subsequently, when my parents now ask, "How's everything?" there's an implied undertone—"Are you *really* OK?" I can't change them, so I just respond as I did before—or attempt to reassure them that "I'm *really* fine."

I prefer knowing the facts about a situation in a straightforward manner—and in that way, am able to best deal with whatever the situation may be. This same attitude applies to my epilepsy. When my seizures surfaced, it drove home the point that there really are gender differences among professionals. Up until the last few years, I hadn't given this much thought, but as I moved from needing an OB-GYN to just needing a gynecologist, this started to move into my consciousness in a nebulous way.

The gender issue, however, was brought into clear focus when I developed epilepsy. I appreciated the forthrightness of my female neurologist and being treated as an intelligent human being, not as the "little lady" by a condescending male physician (the way I was treated several years ago by a male gynecologist, whom I subsequently left). The fact that she readily identified a possible relationship between the seizures and hormonal issues removed whatever angst I might have had.

With my female neurologist, there was an instantaneous comfort level in not having to consider *if* she was making the correct diagnosis or inference, or *really* understood what I was saying. I appreciated dealing with a female professional who understood where I was coming from as a woman. Furthermore, it was particularly helpful that she and her staff provided me with the information regarding possible seizure recurrence and what to look for, possible medication side effects, and so on, that took gender into account.

This approach together with my own research on the Internet gave me a sense of serenity with the circumstances. Since this is a situation that is out of my control—or rather, controlled with medication—so be it.

47

(Age 29) Fortunately, having epilepsy has not affected my family relationships. My family has always been supportive and sensitive to my medical, emotional, and physical needs. Accepting that I have epilepsy has been a work in progress. I was relieved to be given the diagnosis because it answered many of the questions that I had. I was not surprised at all, in fact, and I handled it quite well. My mother, on the other hand, cried in the doctor's office. My friends were supportive but really had no idea what epilepsy was.

Unfortunately, people tend to become nervous because their only exposure is through media and movies, which tend not to depict seizures accurately. More recently, during the last 5 years, I have tried to educate friends, family, and coworkers to reduce their fears.

I wasn't always this open. I never discussed my epilepsy with friends as a teenager because I was embarrassed. There were times when I took my medication only when I felt like it. I was in complete denial. Now, discussing it isn't a problem, probably due to the support I get from the epilepsy clinic and my friends and family.

I have to be very selective when choosing a boyfriend. I cannot have crazy weekends that involve alcohol and little sleep. Whoever I date has to be sensitive to my medical needs. This was very difficult in college, where everyone's world seemed to revolve around alcohol.

My future husband will have to be prepared to be an equal partner in my health care. He will have to be supportive during my pregnancies because there is a higher risk for birth defects. This is a real area of concern for me. I want very much to have happy, healthy children. As a special educator, I have seen the worst-case scenarios and the pros (and sometimes cons) to having a child with special needs. My pediatric neurologist never openly discussed childbearing with me; instead, she would say "We'll cross that bridge when we get to it." This only doubled my fear. I appreciate my new neurologist's honesty and openness.

I have found and learned that, by having epilepsy, one has to be very organized. I cannot become stressed, so that means I cannot wait until the last minute to write that 20-page paper. Some people can pull an all-nighter; my body shuts down whether I want it to or not. Sometimes, I take on too many things with school, work, and social life, and I burn the candle at both ends. If I do not get 8 hours of sleep a day, my body does not function at its optimum level.

The weight factor with my seizure medication has always been difficult. My appetite is extremely high at times—especially before my period, when it is insatiable. If I do not exercise, I can put on a great deal of weight in a short period of time. But when my life is hectic, it is difficult to exercise.

I believe that more educators in the public schools need to learn more about epilepsy. I was surprised to see so many special educators who feared having children with epilepsy in their classrooms. They thought that major changes would have to be made, or they panicked because they did not know how to handle a seizure. I explained that many of the children would just be fatigued and modifications would have to be made for nightly homework or time spent on tiresome projects. They can't believe that I have epilepsy. I almost enjoy telling people just to see the expression on their faces!

48

(Age 59) I have had seizures for the past 7 years that cause disorientation. The seizures have absolutely no effect on my ability to function as a woman, wife, mother, and grandmother on a day-to-day basis. They do, however, have a great effect on my memory. Many things that have happened more than 3 months ago are almost completely erased from my mind. This proves to be most embarrassing when interacting with friends and family. I do, however, have a husband who is both understanding and compassionate and do manage to get through the most important situations without much embarrassment.

My sense of direction is very poor to say the least—in fact, I have none. I have no sense of where houses, streets, etc., are located in relationship to one another. This has affected my independence. I would never attempt to drive a great distance by myself. Whether this situation is a result of my seizures has never been determined, but I do think it is worth mentioning.

Lastly, I must honestly state that the word *epilepsy* is associated with very negative feelings. The very word makes me shudder; associating that word with myself is extremely difficult. I have kept my situation confidential from everybody except, of course, my husband.

I do hope this will help.

49

(Age 39) I think being in high school and having seizures was the hardest part for me. The kids I hung around with said we were all the best of friends. Then one day I had a seizure in school. Soon, I noticed that I didn't have my "best" friends anymore. They still would talk to me, and act very nice, but when they would make plans to go somewhere, they wouldn't call me. One day I asked one of them why. She said they were scared of me.

Back in the early 1970s, nobody ever talked about epilepsy. A lot of people never even heard of it. In high school, all the gossip got around about me, and they started calling me different names like "freak," "half-brain," and "stupid." After a while, I really started feeling like that.

From then on, I didn't feel right about myself. I kept thinking that maybe the seizures were the start or a part of a mental problem for me, and no one could help me. I used to go to bed every night and pray to God just to make me normal like other kids. I'd ask Him, "Why me? What did I do to deserve this?"

All I did was to feel sorry for myself. At that point, I wouldn't say anything to anyone if they didn't know about my seizures. I would just pray I wouldn't have one on a date. But that didn't always work out. Sometimes I would have a seizure, or other times it seemed like everything was going just great for me, until my date would later talk to someone who knew me. They would tell him I had seizures. Then I would be dropped like a hot potato. So I'd go home and cry again: "Why me? Why can't I be normal like other kids?"

Well, after going through this a few times, I gave up for a while. Even so, when no one asked me to my prom, what did I do? Cry again! I felt sorry for myself again!

After I finished high school, I met a nice friend. She didn't know about my problems. She asked me if I wanted a date with one of her brothers. He was 4 years older than me, so I thought I'd give it a chance. Everything went great. We started dating a lot. And, for some reason, I didn't have any seizures around him. Still, I never told him because I was scared he would leave me like all the rest. Our relationship kept getting better, and before you knew it, we were living together.

But the day finally came when he found out. We both went shopping for some food, and right in the middle of one of the aisles, I had a seizure, and he was there for me. When we got back home, he was very upset. That's it! I thought he was going to leave me. But he said the only reason he was upset was because I didn't tell him about my seizures. I told him I loved him and didn't want to lose him, and that's why I never said anything. He told me that what I had was a

Personal Stories

sickness that could be cured. He would never have left me because of that. That made me love him with my whole body, soul, mind, and more. I knew this time I found someone special who would help me and not laugh at me. I felt like I was in paradise.

Not long after that, I found out I was pregnant. We were very happy, but very scared, too. I found out I still had to keep taking all my medication for my seizures. I kept thinking my baby was going to come out addicted, deformed, or born with epilepsy, or maybe even dead. A lot of different thoughts were going through my mind, but everything turned out just great. I had a beautiful little girl.

I asked the doctor to tie my tubes because of my problem, but he refused. He said I was too young. At the time, I was upset and mad! I felt like God gave me a miracle to have a perfect baby. Why take any more chances? Well, without even trying, I found myself pregnant again. Then, the same feelings came back about being happy and scared at the same time. I felt like I was taking my chances with another baby's life, but I guess I am one of the luckiest people, because my second baby girl was just fine, too. This time, I insisted the doctor tie my tubes.

Taking care of my kids was as normal as in any other family. We made it through the "terrible twos," and now my girls are all grown up. They were never scared when I had a seizure, even when they were little. They would sit there and talk to me and hold me, and before you know it, I would come out of my seizure. I have so much love from my family. But, of course, my kids, husband, and I still manage to have our family fights like everyone else.

As our kids grew older, I started getting very depressed because I couldn't find a job on account of my seizures. My husband was working all the time to support all of us. So I went to many nearby neurologists, but they didn't understand how I could have my seizures only when I started my menstrual cycle. They kept telling me one thing had nothing to do with the other. I did find one doctor who said he had no idea why I was having seizures when I started my menstrual cycle, but said he would set up an appointment for me to see a specialist at the university medical center.

Now I feel a lot better, because I know I am talking to doctors who have heard about my situation. These doctors are so nice and really make me feel comfortable. They told me the truth about different medications and different operations. They wanted me to start going to meetings with other people who have epilepsy, because I didn't know anyone else with seizures and felt all alone. I finally did, and felt better because I realized that there were other people out there who had the same problems and questions like "why me?"

So now I know that I am not alone anymore. I also found out what is "normal"; there is not one person on this earth who is perfectly normal. Everyone has problems, but many just keep their problems hidden inside, because they are so scared of what's happening to them. I know that when I found out, I was scared.

But now I know that I'm not alone anymore. That's one thing that has helped me out a lot. There is so much help and understanding that can come from doctors and people when you let them learn about your problems and feelings. No one can help you if you don't help yourself first. Be truthful with your doctor and let him or her know that you are scared. I promise they will help you as best as they can. But you have to take the first step and tell someone.

Sometimes, I think people are scared of epilepsy because they don't know all the facts. They only know what they hear from people or what they might have seen on television. They don't realize there are many different types of seizures and don't take the time to learn about them.

If there is one thing that I have learned after all these years, it's "Don't give up!" If you have a family of your own or are living at home with your parents, you'll end up hurting them more than yourself, because they love you and want the best for you.

Personal Stories

They are not going to give up, and neither should you. That's what you call love.

50

(Age 46) I have never really just sat down to contemplate being a woman with epilepsy. I was not diagnosed until I was in my 40s. Until that time, I just thought I occasionally fainted, though I did also feel something was "wrong" with me.

I was fortunate. My cousin who, coincidentally, is a nurse who specializes in epilepsy, assisted me. She took over and got me to the best doctors and helped me to obtain the best medical care. I cannot imagine what would have happened without her presence.

I *could* say that epilepsy does not affect me. That would be wrong, though. Epilepsy does affect me. I have to be cautious driving, and I have to be sure I get enough sleep and eat properly—all things that are beneficial, anyway.

But I do, at times, feel something is wrong with me, and I know it affects my relationships in many ways. I shy away from any new relationships, partly because I feel once my illness is known, I will probably be abandoned. I did not ask for epilepsy, but I have it, I live with it, and even though it is controlled by medication, I am always aware that it makes me different—not necessarily in a bad way, but different nonetheless.

So I muddle through as best I can. I am still adjusting to being a person with epilepsy. I don't know if it's possible to ever fully adjust; only time will tell. If I could say anything at all to someone else with epilepsy, it would be to get the best medical help you can, and then live your life as best you can. Don't let the epilepsy control you— you control it, and realize this life we have is just one leg of a long journey. Enjoy it as best you can, and know the next leg will be better; of that I am certain.

Epilepsy is a nasty illness, and it should not be allowed to dominate our lives. Also, we should not be ashamed of having epilepsy. We need to ease the stigma associated with it and work toward regaining control over our lives.

51

(Age 40) I started noticing the changes in my late teenage years. Sometimes it felt more like the past than the present. At those times, I knew who I was, but it didn't feel right. Part of me felt like someone else, not the way it should be. I wasn't sure if my mother was really my mother. Her house looked different to me. Things seemed to have a brighter look, and they seemed larger. I felt kind of alone.

I was afraid I might get lost. Sometimes I heard a mean voice laughing inside my head. That sounded wicked. Whenever those feelings came on, I would hold tight to my clothes. I was scared that I might not come out of this feeling.

The feelings kept coming, even after I was married. I would sleep over my mother's house for the 4 days out of the month that these episodes would happen to me. It was always near my period time. I felt like a little girl. I just wanted to be near my mother. I didn't trust anyone, not even my husband.

I was having seizures, but I didn't know it then.

The bad thing was that no one else, including the doctors, knew what was wrong. I went to see a lot of them, and they told me it was nothing but anxiety. It was all in my head, I was told. I used to bring these things on myself, I was told. I went from seeing an internist, to a gynecologist, to a psychiatrist. All they did was to put me on different medicine for nerves. No one ever told me I had seizures.

None of the medicine helped me. They only made me very tired. I just wanted to sleep the whole day. I was very depressed. I wanted to die so many times. I hated living like this the 4 days out of the month.

I never really knew what was going to happen to me. I would never have children, I decided, because I was afraid to. I felt that if I couldn't take care of myself, then I couldn't handle a baby.

Then one night, God answered my prayers. It was about a year ago. My husband saw me in bed at 4:00 a.m., shaking and not responding to him. I bit the inside of my mouth. He got scared and called my parents. They called an ambulance. I was diagnosed as having a grand mal seizure and told I had epilepsy.

I was in the hospital for 3 days. I don't remember any of this. My doctor started me on seizure medicine. My life is now 98% better. I thank God so much for letting me see a good doctor who knows what to do for me. I just started going on small trips with my husband. Right now, I'm not driving because of my seizures, but I have faith some day I will again. I've given up caffeine, coffee, chocolate of all kinds, and tea with caffeine. This has helped me a lot. I miss not having my chocolate, but it's all worth it.

It took 20 years before someone told me I had epilepsy and was having seizures. Now I can say I don't want to die anymore. I want to live, and I love every day.

52

(Age 43) I began having seizures as a complication of viral encephalitis when I was 30 years old. This is something I do not remember, because along with the seizures came memory loss.

My illness had a strong effect on my family. They are still very concerned about all my medications, medical tests, and seizures. My mother (who is now deceased) was always the one who showed the most emotions about my medical condition. Not that the rest of my family didn't care, but it was my mother who seemed to be the most emotional about it.

Since I developed seizures, my relationships with friends have varied. My friends are concerned for me in their own way and do not treat me any different than other people. Unfortunately, it seems as though I have lost friends. I don't blame this on the seizures, just on everyone doing and getting involved in their own thing, which takes up most of their time.

Unfortunately, my independence was taken away from me when I couldn't drive. I had to be dependent on people (mainly my mother, father, and sister) to drive me back and forth to work. I was not able to just get up and go out shopping on my own whenever and wherever I wanted, or, in reality, to go *anywhere* on my own. Sometimes I wonder if this had anything to do with the loss of my friends.

My boyfriend is okay with the epilepsy. His major problem is with the medications I take to try to control the seizures. He sometimes doesn't seem to understand the medication thing—he came into my life approximately 5 years after the encephalitis and never really got to experience the worst of it. He often makes comments like, "You really don't need to take medication." For years, I have tried to get him to come along with me to a doctor's appointment so he could ask questions and make comments, but he just won't.

When I developed epilepsy, my supervisor at work was very understanding and supportive. He was an older gentleman, and I had worked for him for many years. I think he might have understood my situation because his wife had suffered a stroke, and he had gone through a lot with her.

More recently, I was assigned to a new supervisor. I was still able to do the work given to me, but over time I was given less and less work and less and less instruction. There was very little verbal communication between the supervisor and me. Sometimes I don't think the supervisor appreciated the fact that I missed work because of doctor's appointments, medical tests, or just not feeling well after seizures. Soon, I was being outsourced to a couple of other departments; then finally, it progressed to the point that my supervisor wanted to terminate my employment.

I have tried many medications to control my seizures. They have affected me in different ways. Some just didn't help at all, and some made me much too tired. There was one that made me very sexually aroused and two that gave me a very serious rash called *Stevens-Johnson syndrome*. This is something I would not wish on anyone.

It got to the point where there were no more medications that my neurologist could try. Then another neurologist wanted to take me off one medication to try another route. He was definitely taking me off the medication much too quickly—it seemed to have caused me to have a grand mal seizure and made me very discouraged. I ended up going back to the medication I was previously on.

Sometime later, I saw an article about women and epilepsy. I went to see the neurologist who was featured in the article. I then realized that, for the most part, I have my seizures a few days before my period begins. We are now working to see if this observation can lead to treatment that will better control my seizures.

My experiences have taught me that first, and most important, the relationship between patient and doctor is very important. You definitely have to be comfortable with your neurologist. If not, then move on.

53

(Age 19) I've had epilepsy for a little over a year now, and I'm finally learning how to deal with it in a positive way. My cousin has had epilepsy his whole life, and he made it look so easy to live with it.

I had my first seizure when I was at my freshman college orientation. What a great first impression! From that point, I had at least two seizures every month, usually at the same time every month. My mother and I feel it had to do with my menstrual cycle. I still think it does.

I thought that having epilepsy would make me completely different from all of my friends, and that they might feel weird being around me, leaving me alone for most of the time. In fact, over the past year, my best friend and I have become even closer. She has seen all of my seizures, starting with the very first one I had. She is the rock I lean on when I have had an episode, or even when I feel like I'm falling apart.

My relationship with my parents has grown much stronger over this past year and a half than it has been in a long time. I was afraid that even they might think differently of me, or look at me in a different way than they always had. I think since this all started, they *have* looked at me in a different way—a more positive and loving way. They know they don't know how it feels and they can't understand what I'm going through, but they are there to listen and that's all that matters.

It's bad to say this, but I was terrified of what would guys think of this. I was so terrified that I would never find a boyfriend, and if I did, how he would react to me telling him about my epilepsy. To tell you the truth, none of them looked at me any differently than they had without knowing I had epilepsy.

Personal Stories

I think it's only a big deal in your head if you let it be. At first, I thought the world was against me, and I tried to figure out what I did wrong to deserve this. I feel it has made me a much stronger woman than I was before this all happened. It has shown me that I can deal with anything, and that compared to other things in life, this is just a hurdle you have to jump. Once you get over that hurdle, you never have to go back. Once you learn that it will always be with you—and you can accept that—you're set for life.

I think it just takes patience with yourself. I had to understand that immediate results wouldn't happen in one major step. I have now been seizure-free for 7 months—the best thing that's happened to me in over a year. I feel like I have really accomplished something, but it has taken a *lot* of discipline on my part. Being a 19-year-old college student, it's hard not to be able to stay up late with your friends and to take pills on a strict schedule. I've realized I'm not missing out on anything at all, and that this type of discipline and accomplishment has made me feel better about myself and has made me a more confident person.

One year ago, I was told I had epilepsy. I knew it would change my life. I didn't know that it would change it for the better.

54

(Age 39) The sun rises, as do I. With milk in one hand and my morning medication in the other, I watch the world go to work. How I dream to be part of that world again! But my seizures say "no." Seizures have affected many parts of my life. And sometimes they seem to dominate it.

They began 21 years ago, when I was 18 and in college. It was not easy to keep roommates or find the ability to study, but I did it.

After graduating, I started working for a real estate company. I enjoyed this job very much, as well as the many different people I came in contact with. My professionalism, self-confidence, and independence grew greatly during the 13 years I was with the company.

Then, the "day" seizures struck me. Prior to this, all my seizures were at night. Two bad "day" seizures persuaded my boss and a few coworkers that I was no longer good enough to work with them, even after I had received a recent promotion and had brought in a large account. So before they could fire me, I left.

From that time on, my independence has been low. I can't drive, so the world must take me everywhere. Loneliness has become a strong part of my life. It's hard to share or learn from others when people are few and far between. The business world, and all its new and exciting developments, continues without me. If I am ever lucky enough to get a job again in business, will I be able to adapt to all the technological changes?

As a wife, I have been greatly affected by seizures. I never thought I'd find a soul mate because my seizures happen without any warning. But then, God blessed me with Dave, my husband, who is a very caring, loving, and special man. He has done much to put up with my seizures, the many medicines I've tried, and their side effects. My husband carries most of the financial burden. And I feel very guilty about this. I want to work, to earn a true salary to contribute to my family.

Dave worries way too much about me, so much so that sometimes it hurts. For example, if I drop a toothbrush or put a pan in the wrong place, he runs to me, fearing a seizure is occurring. My memory and word recall are declining due to seizures and medication. And with this, my husband's trust in my abilities seems to be declining. This may not be true, and it hurts both of us.

Dave has always wanted children, but I never wanted them. Because there is no warning to my seizures, I felt I could not care well for a child, especially an infant. And I did not want to burden my husband with the "mom" job as well. (He does too much for me already!) After a seizure, I often feel weak and tired through the next day. This would not be good for our child.

My menstrual cycles have been normal, never too painful, and, most often, timely. Seizures have affected me as a sexual partner somewhat. They slow me down and weaken me; often, making love must be postponed. But the quality of our sexual lives is still good.

I have always felt myself to be a good friend; however, seizures have demolished my self-confidence to be a good friend to someone else. Because I can no longer easily visit a friend, it is hard for me to give assistance whenever needed. I offer, but many times cannot come through. Since I am alone so much, I sometimes get too excited when I am about to visit a friend. This anticipation does me in, and I have a seizure.

Losing my memory has hurt many aspects of my life. I am unable to remember names, finish sentences, and recall places that I've been to. This demands a great deal from my friends, family, and husband, especially patience. I do have a few special friends who have patience and have cared for me a long time—I know they won't give up on me.

Seizures have affected my life, more so as I get older. But as my husband continues to say, "You can't give up trying. There is an answer somewhere."

I pray to God every single day the answer will be found.

55

(Age 42) I have only had three grand mal seizures and don't feel like my life has gone through major changes. However, during the 6-month period that I had these three seizures, my family did have several issues to deal with.

My two children, aged 9 and 13, were with me when I had the seizures. They thought I was dying, that they were losing their mother forever. My 9-year-old son ended up with post-traumatic stress syndrome and was in counseling for 6 months. My 13-year-old daughter became withdrawn until she studied and read everything I could find for her on seizures and epilepsy. (There was hardly anything age-appropriate at the time.) Only after she learned about seizures was she able to start working through her fears.

I was more concerned for my children and how this affected them than I was for myself. I believe this is a major concern for most mothers with epilepsy. We put ourselves on the back burner to help our loved ones first. This must be very frustrating for our doctors.

I was put on medication but could not deal with the side effect of fatigue; it is very difficult to be a mom and be so tired. I was then put on another drug but had to go off because of FDA problems or something. Then I went on yet another medication, but after 9 months I had a severe problem with my pancreas and gallbladder, and was taken off the drug and put on the medication I was on in the first place.

A major result of all these medication changes was loss of time. The amount of time that it takes to go through with doctor appointments and lab work is unbelievable. It was not something I really thought about or even realized. Then one day, as I was going out the door, my son asked me, "Doesn't it bug you to have to go to the doctor's so much?" Alert to my child's needs—remember, he comes first—I said, "It must seem like I'm always going to a doctor's office. Are you worried when I do?" This conversation was a good opening to talking about how I was doing and whether my son (age 16) was still concerned. Bottom line, he'd like me to be perfect, no health problems at all, but he's glad I do what I should to take care of myself. And even though it seems like a lot of time is involved, he thinks it's worth it.

There have been no major changes for me in employment or independence. My relationships with friends haven't really been affected, since they know I take antiseizure medicine and they do not treat me any differently.

My husband and I are close and supportive of one another. The only thing that we are wrestling with at this moment is the decision about whether I should go off antiseizure medicine. He wants me to take it for the rest of our lives. He only saw one seizure, but he never wants to see me go through that again. And there's a puzzle... because I don't "go through it," I don't even remember it—I don't even get an aura—so really, he is the one who "goes through it." And I don't want him to.

But at the age of 42, it's hard to think of being on a medication for the next 40 years. This is why it's important for women with epilepsy to have a good doctor (like I do) to help them with their concerns and fears. I had a very nice (and seemingly competent) neurologist tell me that I had no reason to be worried about my medication causing bone loss long term, that there was no connection; he patted me on the head and sent me on my way. The weight of medical evidence disagrees. Women have an obligation to themselves and their loved ones to make sure their doctors are well rounded in all aspects of epilepsy and the medicines that are used, so they can live normal, happy lives.

It's hard to think of myself as having epilepsy, but I have had seizures. I would not like to have them again. My family and I know that if I should have more seizures, it will be all right. We can take care of it and can learn how to deal with *whatever* comes our way.

56

(Age 31) I've lived two-thirds of my life as a person with epilepsy. The original diagnosis was "idiopathic tonic-clonic epilepsy, onset at puberty." And it's *epilepsy*, damn it, not *seizure disorder*. I *hate* the term *seizure disorder*! It makes me feel abnormal, somehow wrong or shameful.

Epilepsy is a part of who I am, an integral part of my identity. I don't know if I'd give it up—you know, have surgery for it. The idea of someone digging around in my brain freaks me out, and what if it changed me? Like when I went off a seizure medication once, and found out how much of my depression was due to the drug. Ten years of thinking I knew who I was . . . gone with a single medication change. It's not likely to ever be an issue again; my seizures are well controlled with another drug.

I want to have one or more children, hopefully in the near future. This will mean considering the effects of hormonal changes on me, the possible effects of medication on the fetus (it turns out that the blood barrier between a mother and the child in the womb is often more than sufficient), issues around nursing the baby, and lack of sleep.

It's weird that something so intimate and so comfortable for me scares other people so. Most don't even know there are different types of seizures. It's physically impossible to swallow your own tongue, people! I have the best-known type of seizure, the type everyone thinks of when they hear the word epilepsy. I flop like a fish out of water.

I tell my friends what to do and what not to do if I seize while around them: *not* to call an ambulance, to get me somewhere dark and quiet with a can of Coke and a couple of aspirin, and to leave me there for 15 minutes or so. Their job is to make sure I don't hit my head on something. They aren't to put anything in my mouth, and aren't to hold me still or drag me into a prone position. And that they're not to worry if I bleed from the mouth, or if I can't talk right afterwards; it's just my bitten tongue.

I also tell them about status epilepticus and what to do if I go into it. That I have never had it, and that the chance that they'll ever see me seize during the day is very, very small. I haven't had a daytime seizure in over 10 years. On the other hand, nothing has ever controlled my nocturnal seizures. I only know when I have them because I do a tongue check every morning.

I've been told that I see and say things during a seizure. I never remember it, but the very idea fills me with wonder and joy. A historical overview: in some cultures, I would have been made a shaman; in some, considered holy; in some, burnt for being possessed; in others, given medication so no one had to know.

When I was a teenager, it made me angry when my mom would say I had a physical disability. It was just something I had. It took me years to wean her off her habit of periodically checking up on me when I took a bath.

Then the Americans with Disabilities Act happened, and suddenly I was disabled and protected. Except nothing really changed. The ADA is great, as long as you have a visible and obvious disability, the type where all it takes is one look to see it—the type where everyone automatically pities you, and stares at you on public transportation.

But most people with epilepsy don't wear a helmet. If your disability is invisible, then the ADA doesn't go nearly far enough. It should have done away with the "preexisting condition" clause in health insurance.

It's a wall, always waiting around the next corner to slam me in the face. *That's* the most disabling part of having epilepsy.

57

(Age 49) I am a woman with epilepsy who has recently reached menopause. Because my epilepsy was influenced by hormonal factors in the past, I am wondering what effect menopause will have on my seizures now. I also question what effects my epilepsy and my medications will have on my menopause. Does menopause last longer in women with epilepsy? I know stress has a lot to do with seizure activity, and that stress can be a part of menopause because of all the change in bodily function. Any connection? Should I take hormone replacement therapy (HRT)? Would HRT have an impact on my seizure activity? Would my seizure medications work with HRT? I've been reading a lot about natural hormone replacement (NHR). Perhaps I should try this route. Would NHR work with my medications OK?

Women with epilepsy everywhere who are reaching this stage in life are asking these questions. Unfortunately, there aren't many answers yet.

Five years ago, I had a right temporal lobectomy. I lived with horrible complex partial seizures for 14 years, sometimes reaching up to 15 seizures a month. Although it took a while, I am now down to about one or two nocturnal partial seizures every few months. I can live with that! Between the surgery and a new medication, my life is so much better; however, in all the reading I've done so far on epilepsy and menopause, I've not seen anything regarding women who have undergone surgery for their seizures in the past. More questions... Will my brain surgery have an effect on my menopause? I guess the research just isn't there yet.

With the way things have been going for me, I'm not sure I want to "rock the boat." I don't want difficult seizure activity to reenter my life. So do I just sit back and let the sweat drip? Hot flashes are not the most pleasant things to deal with: I get the rush and *boom*! I better sit down, as I often get dizzy and short of breath. I remove whatever clothing is appropriate for the moment and fan myself with a souvenir from New Orleans, which I now keep with me at all times! Then there are the night sweats, another wonderful experience. My poor husband is always waking up in

Personal Stories

the middle of the night freezing, as I have thrown all the covers off the bed!

What about the questions of breast cancer, heart problems, osteoporosis, and memory loss (although the latter is a given for me because of the seizures, the medications, the brain surgery, and age)? Would HRT or NHR work with me regarding these questions? Oh, perhaps I should just say the heck with it all. Our foremothers made it through without all this fuss. But how many of them had epilepsy?

Recently, I hooked myself up with an epilepsy specialist. He knows all about epilepsy, hormones, and how we women work, and he has an open mind. I decided to check in with him regarding my menopause and how best to deal with it. I figured he could help walk me through this stage of my life, rather than a gynecologist who probably doesn't know a great deal about epilepsy and its many facets. Two years ago, when I just began having a few night sweats, my old GYN wanted to slap the patch onto me without taking any hormone tests or without taking my epilepsy into consideration. See you later! I'm with a new GYN now. I hope to get my two new doctors hooked up.

Then there is my husband, God bless him. He has been to hell and back with me through all the years of seizures, brain surgery, and then recovery. He stood by me every step of the way. He is so happy the complex partial seizures are gone, hopefully for good. I know he is concerned regarding all the questions surrounding my menopause. He wants what is best for me, but certainly does not want to see the heavy seizure activity return.

You know, through it all, I think the most frustrating part for him has been my difficulty with memory. Between the seizures, the medications, the surgery, and now menopause, my memory has not been the best—shall we say it's a bit hampered? It drives him crazy when I ask him a question over again that he just answered a few moments ago. I know it really bothers him when I can't recall the lovely dinner we had a while back at that beautiful restaurant. It hurts him that I have difficulty remembering other places we've been and things we've done together. When he gives me a few clues, sometimes I can bring certain memories back.

He is always reminding me of things because he knows I'll just forget: "Take your medications. Do you have your keys, your glasses, your coat? Did you bring your medications?" God, he is wonderful. Do you know that ever since my brain surgery, he brings me my morning medicine with a glass of water at the exact same time every day?! Because he knows that otherwise, I'll just forget to take them. My faded memory function is frustrating for us both. I don't like having to be reminded of everything. It stinks. Still, he has stuck with me through it all.

I guess love must really have something to do with it.

58

(Age 56) I am a 56-year-old woman, and although I have been engaged three times, I never married. My reasons for ending these and other relationships were many, though there was one reason that was true for all: they all wanted to see me or be around me too much and that made me feel smothered. I had to get out.

I realize now that I need a lot of space and solitude in my life. I believe one effect of my seizures is that I can only take so much stimulation, and then I need to be off by myself somewhere where it is quiet. It's like my brain needs to shut down and be restored by solitude; actually, I need so much it worries me. This makes me think of my father, who disappeared for long periods of time throughout my life. He was well educated, highly sensitive, and an alcoholic. I remember at times seeing his eyeballs roll upwards in his head, and he could be found muttering, or at least moving his lips, at other times. I think he may have had seizures and self-medicated with alcohol. His need to disappear may be just like my need to shut down and seek seclusion and silence. I have lived alone in my own home for almost 22 years.

I spent over 20 years practicing many kinds of meditation, including chanting. The benefits were wonderful in terms of being able to feel centered and connected to the ground. As time went on, I lacked the discipline to keep at it, but I think it could possibly replace medication. I wish I had the will to keep at it. Maybe someday!

I have always enjoyed sex, but at times I seemed to equate sex with death and afterwards would feel a profound sadness, which frightened me. I think that could be why, in retrospect, I myself abused alcohol at one time. I am working on this issue of sex, death, and relationships with a psychiatrist.

I have never thought about having children, and I don't know why. I did teach first through ninth grade for almost 14 years. I enjoyed the children, learned a great deal about them, and am very happy for the experience. The truth is, I do not think I ever had the psychic or physical energy to care for children, and I have always felt so fragmented. It is so difficult for me to get through a day that I cannot imagine having children.

I was diagnosed 10 years ago with epilepsy. I feel dissociated a lot, and that makes relationships difficult. My seizures are so experiential that I could never talk about them with family or friends, and that is a true hardship. I have spoken to other people with similar seizures, which is like finding an old army buddy to share old wartime experiences, but some of their experiences have frightened me, too.

My seizures make me feel that I am different from everyone else—kind of like odd man out, maybe even mysterious. I feel very sad about them and think it is my fault. Sometimes I ask myself, "What's wrong with you?" Actually, I often heard those words when I was growing up. Maybe that's why I am so analytical.

I smell burning rubber or a skunk fairly often. I've long since stopped asking if anyone else does. My nervous system, which I call my "lining," is jumpy, wiry, or tense pretty much most of the time, but it sure is nice when things settle down inside me. Sometimes I think the inside of me comes outside and moves along just ahead of me. How about that one? I bet someone out there knows just what I mean.

Relationships are difficult because I can lose my train of thought midsentence or forget what I was trying to say halfway through. I am almost afraid to discuss a book or movie; I have to think it out thought by thought. The thoughts don't carry themselves anymore. It makes me feel stupid.

Sometimes, if I put myself on what I call "high alert" and get things out by spoonful, so to speak, I come off all right. I am afraid people won't want to be around me, or they will think something is wrong with me. I make comments in small doses, and nobody knows that I am feeling too scattered to continue.

As a social worker, I interview people and assess their eligibility for particular programs. This is difficult, because I have to disseminate so much information. Some days are not good. I feel embarrassed and stupid when I stutter or forget things, and there are long pauses before I speak. Fortunately, this is not always the case, and I have my little tricks of getting the clients to read and do some of the writing.

I am on hormone replacement therapy now. I have lots of seizures in a cyclical pattern. I feel excessive excitability, nervousness, a symphony of headaches, and roller coaster emotional swings during these seizure times. I have days when I cannot sit still, and I jump from one thing to another, finishing none, and also days when I need to urinate about every 15 to 20 minutes, round the clock.

I work part-time now, 6 hours a day, and it is getting to be a bit too long for me. I have a wonderful supervisor who knows a bit about my seizures and me, and this makes me feel relaxed at work. I also work in a very laid-back environment, though my work can be demanding. I have had this job going on 10 years. I am underemployed and sometimes feel ashamed about this, but on the plus side, it is easy there to go blank midsentence, forget, and have days when I do a lot of staring. I am comfortable among my coworkers. I can interact as much as I want. I have my own office, which is wonderful for my "off" days.

If I can get myself to slow down, almost to slow motion, I function better. I do feel wonderfully happy at times. I have developed a sensitivity to others and enormous empathy, somehow, for the elderly. I guess I feel their fragility, but in a different way. Because of my epilepsy, I am more caring, sympathetic, and insightful. I pick up vibrations about people and trust my intuition completely. Maybe that's a bonus! That makes me feel good about myself.

59

(Age 30) My epilepsy started when I was 2 years old. Since I have been having periods, my seizures usually occur near the start of my menstrual cycle. My periods, however, have been getting further and further apart. To me, that is due to my medicine.

My seizures prevent me from driving and limit my social activities and independence; however, I am presently in the process of exploring medical options for my condition, like surgery and a nerve stimulator. If these treatments were successful, I would perhaps become seizure-free and able to drive.

60

(Age 39) I was diagnosed with epilepsy as a child. After being started on a combination of medications, my seizures were controlled. I didn't really think about my epilepsy as I grew up. It didn't affect my daily activities, and at times, I forgot I had it.

My family relationships were never affected. There was a difference of opinion between my Mom and Dad as to how much I should be told. My Dad thought that I should not tell anyone about my seizures or that I was on medication; it followed, then, that my Dad wouldn't let me sleep over at other kids' houses since my seizures were nocturnal and he was concerned about people finding out. My Mom, on the other hand, was the one who told me that I had epilepsy, and for that I am grateful.

I have a few close friends and coworkers, and I have been very open about my seizure history with them. This has not affected my friendships in any way.

My epilepsy was brought to the forefront again after I was married and began to think about having children. I had to be aggressive with my neurologist about tapering off one of my medications, since that particular medication could affect the fetus. My Dad was very resistant to any medication changes because I was seizure-free. I tapered off without any problem and was able to get pregnant easily. At that time, I began my association with the university epilepsy center. I felt it was important to have all my physicians within one institution for better communication during my pregnancy.

I had a healthy baby boy without any seizure reoccurrence, and went on to have another baby 19 months later, again, without any problems. There was close monitoring of both pregnancies for any birth defects and a close eye on my drug levels throughout my pregnancies.

I have been seizure-free for over 20 years and my dilemma is whether to stay on my medication or taper off and see what happens. Because my children are young and there would be driving restrictions if I had seizures, I have decided to stay on my medication. My other concern is what affect menopause will have on my seizure history.

I am also careful to watch over the children for any seizure activity—none so far.

In my case, epilepsy has not prevented me from accomplishing much in my life. I graduated from college, trained to be a nurse, became a wife, and experienced motherhood. Hopefully, sharing these few reflections may help or inspire you.

61

(Age 26) I think I have desired independence since my high school years. Back then, I would say to myself, "I am not going to get married until I am 32 years old, like Mom did. I want to live my life and prove that I can be somebody without the help of someone else."

Mom and Dad had always felt that their child—female especially—*needed* their help; and so I grew up needing their solutions and wisdom, but got spoiled and a little naïve about how to function in the world. How was I supposed to learn if I always depended on them?

Then I met a very nice guy in college; I'll call him Frank. He didn't give two toots about my seizures, even though I scared the other students and made my teacher think I was faking or taking illegal drugs. Frank saw me fall down, cry, and act drunk because of my medications, but he told jokes to make me laugh. I knew we'd make plans soon for marriage, but my parents wouldn't let us live together. They had me by a hook—the same hook I'd been on for years—insurance. I needed to live in their household so that I could receive medical coverage. Frank and I rolled our eyes at that one, but eventually got married anyway. I wish I'd waited to get married, but knew I couldn't, or was afraid that he'd walk away.

So why'd I get married? I knew that I'd be very lucky to find another nice man like him and I was afraid of being off of insurance. It scared me. I'm working to get a job that will get me insurance coverage, in case the inevitable occurs and Frank and I part ways.

My periods have gone from 28 days (age 15) to 23 days (now). Is this hormone-related?

I still feel bits and pieces of desire for my husband and am working on building up our sex life. Since we've been married, we've only had sex three times in 3 years. I'm only 26. It hurts to have him put his penis in me, and I feel like my opening has shrunken—I understand this is common in women with epilepsy. Ouch.

I used to feel very guilty about this, and probably still do. I know it's not me, it's my medications. I love him. He loves me, and wouldn't leave me because of piddly sexual desires. He's like that.

Neither of us wants kids right now. It's a nice idea, but kids are too much work. I'd like to live a little with my loved one. I know I *can* have them, so I'm not worried.

I've been asked twice to leave the job I was hired for. I was young, and so I complied. Then I was hired to welcome and talk to visitors at a museum. When I told the manager about my seizures, she exclaimed, "Why didn't you tell us you had them?!" She changed my position. I was forced to sit at a ticket booth so I wouldn't "fall."

I told her that the beeping of cash registers and being in a hot ticket booth (plus being bored out of my mind) would induce seizures. She shrugged. After 3 weeks and a couple of seizures, I quit. I learned that while it's OK to have diabetes, keel over from a heart attack on the job, or be addicted to cigarettes and spend as much time as possible smoking them on the job, *no one* wants to have or *learn* how to deal with a person with epilepsy.

How do I get by? I am usually pretty upbeat, and I believe in myself and in a positive God in the sky. When I'm down, which occurs sometimes after a seizure, song lyrics especially bring the light back to my eyes.

62

(Age 33) I've had seizures since birth. From what I understand, the first seizure I had was a grand mal seizure. Nearly all the seizures I had after that were petit mal. I'm not really sure how many seizures I had each month up until the eighth grade because I didn't personally keep track of them. When I was a freshman in high school, I tried to keep track of my seizures. During my 4 years of high school, I usually had four to five seizures a month, though there were a few months I had eight to ten seizures. On some of the days that I had seizures, I was able to stay at school and do what I had planned to do because I felt OK.

After I graduated from high school, my seizures did cut back a little bit. I went to the doctor and had some tests for my epilepsy. We found out that my seizures came from both sides of my brain. I had a lot of changes made in my medications. I don't remember the reasons I went off any of them except for one, which made me tired and lose my appetite. It was a very uncomfortable time for me. I was in pain for hours after eating—a very sharp pain. After I stopped taking this medication, it took about 4 to 6 years for my appetite to come back.

For the past couple years, I've been seeing a different doctor. We've tried a few other medications, including a long-acting form of one of my old medications. Despite this, I had a grand mal seizure this year. I was at a friend's house and scared both her and her son. I had to go to the hospital to have the seizure stopped, and was there for 29 hours before being released. I was told the seizure came on because the blood level of my seizure medication was low.

Recently, I had a stimulator put in my chest that connects to a nerve in the left side of my neck. Nine days after the surgery I had a grand mal seizure, but it wasn't set to handle a strong seizure yet.

Now it's just a matter of time to see if it will work for me to control my seizures better.

63

(Age 33) Like so many others, my epilepsy began in adolescence. I was approximately 13 years old when I had my first seizure, though I was not diagnosed until the age of 15. In fact, the reason I was not diagnosed was because I was unaware I was having seizures.

I was having a type of seizure called *myoclonic seizures.* What I experienced were small jerks of my limbs that occasionally would "trip me up." I just thought I was a klutz, and so didn't report these incidents to anyone. Furthermore, at that time in my life, I had only known one other person to have a seizure, my oldest brother. He had grand mal seizures, which is the type of seizure people typically think about when they hear the term *epilepsy*, and I was no exception to that rule.

For these reasons, the first time I ever visited a doctor's office about my seizure disorder was only after I had my first grand mal (tonic-clonic) seizure.

During my doctors' visits, I encountered many children with epilepsy but not anyone my age. I often thought how nice it would have been to have had the opportunity to talk with other teens my age, especially girls, about epilepsy—to have shared our experiences with each other, to know that there were others like me struggling with the same issues. So, often times, during my teen years, I felt isolated, even though intellectually I knew I wasn't alone.

Furthermore, when I was diagnosed, my doctor told me I had a low threshold to seizures, and that this meant I had a "seizure disorder." The word *epilepsy* was never mentioned.

My brother, David, is 11 years older than I am. His seizures had gone into remission by the time of my first seizure. He "grew out of them," as they say. While no one in my family was ever embarrassed or ashamed of David's epilepsy, it wasn't something we talked about much. David's seizures were well controlled. It wasn't a big deal.

But still, I knew what my brother had was called *epilepsy*. So when the doctors told me I had a seizure disorder, I just figured that epilepsy and seizure disorders might somehow be related but were not the same thing. I was young, and I didn't ask many questions.

But it wasn't until college that I discovered, through my own research, that *epilepsy* is simply an umbrella term for *seizure disorder*—that they were, in fact, synonymous. Can you imagine how silly I felt? But I also felt betrayed. Why hadn't the doctors just told me I had epilepsy? Why didn't they explain that seizure disorder and epilepsy were the same? And why hadn't my parents said anything?

Looking back, the one question that was uppermost in my mind was whether or not I would have this for the rest of my life, and to be honest, I don't recall whether I asked that question or not. In any event, the answer would probably have been, "You'll probably grow out of it," like my brother.

The answer was different when I was rediagnosed, years after that first doctor's visit, with juvenile myoclonic epilepsy. This is a form of epilepsy that is genetic in origin and is lifelong. This type of epilepsy is characterized by the fact that it first occurs in adolescence with myoclonic jerks, which may occur for a year or two before tonic-clonic seizures usually begin. My situation was very typical.

It was during this visit that I was told I would not outgrow my seizures. The likelihood that I would have epilepsy for the rest of my life devastated me. What about children? Could I have them? What did all this mean?

Until I became active in a Women and Epilepsy program, it never occurred to me that my seizures and menstrual cycle might somehow be connected. Perhaps I just wasn't as in tune with my body as other women—again, that feeling of complete stupidity. How could I miss that? How could I not know? And, if I had known, would it have made a difference? Would my doctor have believed me?

What I realize now is that hormone-sensitive seizures are not an uncommon experience for women with epilepsy. I also know that one of the most common experiences women face is doubt from their physicians about this connection.

I now know that my seizures will last my entire life. I also know that I have monthly myoclonic seizures just before and during my menstrual cycle. I am in the process of reevaluating the medications I am currently taking, in the hopes that we can control the myoclonic seizures. Unfortunately, as I grow older, I tend to have more breakthrough tonic-clonic seizures. The reason for this is, as yet, unknown. I suspect that it has a lot to do with stress.

Even though I have epilepsy and face a lifetime of unknowns, I do know one thing: I am a better person for my experiences. I am not afraid of life, and I fully intend to have a family of my own.

My epilepsy has made me committed to the cause of epilepsy and to advocating for the improved quality of life of all people with epilepsy. But I will always hold a special place in my heart for the over 1 million women and girls with epilepsy in the United States who have been and will continue to deal with the very unique issues of being a woman with epilepsy.

64

(Age 37) How many men does it take to change a light bulb? One—but the job will never get done. How many women does it take to change a light bulb? Many—but they will find the problem, make a plan, and get it done today. And they will work together while doing so!!

How can we apply this riddle to our own lives with epilepsy? It means that if you have concerns about your health or the impact of your epilepsy on others, then you need to find out what the problem is, get help from others, find out the necessary information, figure out the problem, and address it!

You won't be able to do it alone. I suspect that many of you have tried, and felt that you didn't get anywhere, that no one heard your concerns or knew what to do. The "light bulb" didn't get fixed.

Why? Any number of reasons, but let's start by looking at ourselves. What do we know about "our bodies and ourselves"? Are women's health issues important to you?

I asked these questions of myself not long ago, and in finding the answer, looked back into my past to see what I knew about having epilepsy and being a woman, and when I knew it. Let me share this journey with you.

I was diagnosed with a possible seizure disorder when I was 7 years old, but the seizures probably actually began when I was 1 year old. Of course, no one was quite sure that they were seizures, and luckily, they were infrequent enough that my parents felt safe just watching for a while to see if the events would go away or "declare themselves."

Well, they declared themselves, and I was placed on medicine. Over the years, I tried coming off medication many times. I am one of the lucky ones in that medicine controls the outward manifestations of my seizure disorder; however, I am one of the unlucky ones who need to continue medicines indefinitely.

When I was an adolescent, I had some breakthrough seizures. Why? I don't know. Maybe they were related to growth spurts, or perhaps due to the hormone changes of puberty. No one even thought about the connection between hormones and seizures in the "olden" days, so I can't be sure. Interestingly, I also had irregular and painful menstrual periods; of course, so did many teenage girls, but was there a connection with my seizures? Doctors didn't know. My challenge was to find a gynecologist who would listen and help. This search has lasted a long time.

The first one tried all sorts of pain medicines and birth control pills. He even told me, a 16-year-old girl, to get pregnant in order to fix the problems with my menstrual period! He never asked me about my seizures or my medicines. He never explained that the birth control pills would not be effective for contraception, and I never knew that breakthrough bleeding was a sign I should watch for. I was a naïve girl with seizures that I did not understand, taking medicines that I did not understand, either.

I did not understand my body and what I was dealing with. I wasn't given the information about my hormonal status, but then,

Personal Stories

I didn't ask! I was told some information about my seizures, but chose not to hear it or believe it. I complained about taking my medicine and blamed my parents, especially my mother, but I didn't take responsibility for my epilepsy for a long time.

I was in denial. I don't think that I accepted that I had seizures until I was in college, and I didn't understand what I really needed to know until many years later.

A turning point came when I had a cluster of breakthrough seizures as a young adult. Finally, I was able to get all the latest information in my hands. Scientific and technological advances had been made: there were more sophisticated EEGs, improved methods for imaging the brain, and both the capability and desire to evaluate the hormonal aspects of a woman's body. Doctors were thinking about the relationships of hormones to brain function.

Wow! What a difference. In many ways it was exciting, and in many other ways, very scary. Knowledge can be unsettling because once you have it, you need to digest what it means, for better or for worse, and figure out what to do with it. This is a daunting challenge for anyone.

I learned that I did have hormonal disturbances that likely had a connection to my seizures and my history of menstrual irregularities. I also learned about birth control pills and their appropriate use. I found out that I may have difficulty getting pregnant, but if this were true, that there were some things that could be done. That was fantastic information because I, like many other women, was under the mistaken perception that I may not be able to have children at all!

Now armed with a better understanding of my situation, I became overwhelmed. What did all this mean? What was I going to have to go through to have kids? Maybe I really couldn't. If hormones affected my seizures, would my seizures get worse if I became pregnant? And if so, how would I continue to work? The list of questions and worries grew longer, and I am sure that many of you have thought about these issues at some point. I only came up with more questions as I learned more about seizures and hormonal function.

And to make matters even more confusing, I received different answers from different doctors and friends. It soon became clear to me that neither the scientific community, of which I am a member, nor society at large had all the answers. There were a few answers, but they were incomplete.

I needed to learn to deal with the inconsistencies and incompleteness of our understanding. I also started to think about other women who didn't have access to the expert care and research that I did. It just wasn't fair and acceptable to me anymore.

I decided that I needed to do something to change this. That's why I became active in the development of a program for women with epilepsy in my community. If these issues are important to you, seek out the experts in *your* community and get involved!

Glossary

Americans with Disabilities Act (ADA): A federal law that protects the rights of physically or mentally challenged people.

Aura: A seizure that consists of a sensation or motor movement without loss of consciousness.

Complex partial seizure: A seizure that disrupts a portion of the brain's electrical activity, resulting in loss of conscious contact with others or surroundings.

Convulsion: A seizure involving massive involuntary contractions and jerks of the muscles in association with loss of consciousness. This is the clonic phase of a tonic-clonic seizure.

CT scan: Computed tomography. A CT machine uses X-rays to produce photographs of different parts of the body.

EEG: Electroencephalogram. A recording of the brain's electrical activity.

EKG: Electrocardiogram. A recording of the heart's electrical activity.

Encephalitis: Inflammation of the brain that is usually due to infection and that may cause epilepsy.

Endocrinologist: A physician who specializes in the diagnosis and treatment of disorders of the glands (also called the *hormonal system*, it includes the pituitary, thyroid, and adrenal glands).

Epilepsy: The tendency to have recurrent seizures from known or unknown causes.

Estrogen: A female sex hormone produced in the ovaries.

FDA: U.S. Food and Drug Administration.

Fetus: The developing human life that grows in the uterus (womb) of a pregnant woman.

Folate: A form of folic acid.

Folic acid: A water-soluble B vitamin that may play an important role in fetal development.

Grand mal seizure: *See* Tonic-clonic seizure.

Idiopathic: No known cause.

Internist: A physician who specializes in the diagnosis and treatment of adults with nonsurgical or nonobstetric disorders.

Menses: The periodic (usually monthly) discharge of blood through the vagina from a nonpregnant uterus.

Menstrual cycle: A regular period of time, usually approximately 28 days, during which an egg develops in the ovary and is then released. The cycle ends (or begins, depending on one's point of view) with the menses.

MRI: Magnetic resonance imaging. An MRI machine uses magnetic forces to generate pictures of various body parts.

Neural tube defect: A birth defect involving the spinal column and sometimes the spinal cord.

Neuroendocrinologist: A physician trained in the diagnosis and treatment of disorders involving the interactions between the hormonal system and the nervous system.

Neurologist: A physician who specializes in the diagnosis and treatment of disorders of the nervous system (brain, spinal cord, and nerves).

Neuropathy: A disorder, usually progressive, of the nerves in the arms and legs (known as the *peripheral nerves*).

Obstetrician-gynecologist (OB-GYN): A physician trained specifically to deliver babies and to treat diseases of the female reproductive organs and tissues (uterus, ovaries, vagina, and breasts).

Partial seizure: A seizure that disrupts a part of the brain's electrical activity.

Period: Slang for *menses.*

Petit mal seizures: An old term for either absence or complex partial seizures. Refers to episodes of staring and unresponsiveness.

Premenstrual syndrome: Symptoms that are experienced before the menses; may include bloating, weight gain, anxiety, and moodiness.

Progesterone: A female sex hormone produced in the ovaries during the second half of the menstrual cycle that prepares the uterus for receiving the fertilized egg.

Puberty: The period of life during which adult physical and sexual characteristics develop and the capability for sexual reproduction is attained.

Seizure: A sudden disruption of the brain's electrical activity. The main symptom of epilepsy.

Status epilepticus: Seizure activity that is continuous for 30 minutes or more. Status epilepticus is a medical emergency and an ambulance should be called. One should suspect status epilepticus if a tonic-clonic seizure has lasted for more than 5 minutes.

Stevens-Johnson syndrome: A severe and sometimes fatal syndrome of flulike symptoms and skin lesions that vary from blisters to loss of skin from all body areas. The lesions also involve the lining of the mouth.

Temporal lobe epilepsy: A form of epilepsy in which seizures arise from the temporal lobe.

Titration (of medication): Adjustment, usually an increase in dosage, of medication under a doctor's supervision.

Tonic-clonic seizure: A seizure, previously called *grand mal*, in which the person suddenly loses consciousness, becomes stiff, and has massive involuntary contractions and jerks of the muscles.

Glossary

Index

acceptance, 14–15, 17, 62, 81
  by boyfriend, 18
  of depression, 63
  of diagnosis, 17, 60, 85
  difficulty of parents, 11
  of parent with epilepsy, by children,
    7, 59
  by families, 46, 57, 80
  by friends, 5, 57
  by husband, 37, 76
  by self, 15, 17, 38, 60, 63, 85–86, 98, 103
  by suitemate, 41
accommodations
  courtship discussions about, 52
  by friends, 53
  during sex, 50
  in workplace, 52
admission of epilepsy
  difficulties with, 3–4
  fear of, 2–3
  response variety, 14

adopting children, 19, 75
alcohol abuse, 69–70, 108
Americans With Disabilities Act, 27,
    50, 104
ammonia smells, 9
anticonvulsant medication, 17
appetite, and medication, 87,
    114–115
automobile accident, 52–53

balance difficulties, 10, 40, 47
blackout experience, 9, 24–25

chanting, 107
children
  adoption of, 19, 75
  concerns of husbands, 21, 32
  coping with seizures of, 13–14
  deciding for/against, 13, 19–20, 21–22
  healthy, success in having, 17
  support of parent with epilepsy by, 17

cognitive function, and medication, 10, 58
communication issues, 50, 51
concerns
    of children, for parent with epilepsy, 57
    of employers, 56
    of friends, 95
    for others, 4, 17
    of parents, 18, 26, 101, 111
    of pregnancy, 21–22, 86
    of spouse, 106
    of sudden seizure, 65, 78
confidence
    of friends, 49
    in having children, 23
    influence on emotional security, 17
    loss of, 55
    of parents, 21
    in self, 50, 67–68, 73, 99–100
coworkers
    lack of support from, 99
    support from, 67, 86, 110

dating issues, 43, 51, 78, 89
    difficulties of teens, 15
    fear of discovery, 68
    hiding of epilepsy, 46, 68
    revelation of epilepsy, 2, 14, 17, 54
    sensitivity to medical needs, 86
denial, 86, 120
depression
    acceptance of, 63
    from employment difficulties, 90
    from having seizures, 75, 79
    from not driving, 60
    relief through counseling, 12
    as side effect of medicine, 103
    from suicide of husband, 81
diagnosis
    acceptance of, 17, 60, 85
    in childhood, 111
    life-changing influence of, 64
    openness about, 67
    for pharmacologic treatment, 11
    sense of relief from, 18, 86
    spousal reaction to, 76

difficulties
    with admission of illness, 3–4
    dealing with fears, 65
    with driving, 8, 10, 13, 23, 66–67
    of families, with acceptance, 11–12
    having children, 20
    maintaining employment, 38
    from memory loss, 109
    of spouses, 6
disorientation, 64, 87
divorce, 2, 37
doctors
    attitudes/advice regarding pregnancy, 7, 66, 75, 78, 90
    "doctorese" speak by, 44
    encouragement by, 38
    following advice of, 37, 90
    gratefulness for, 23
    helpfulness of, 34, 38, 90, 94, 102
    nonhelpfulness/nonreassurance from, 19, 38, 54
    support from, 16, 41
    trustworthiness of, 16
    truthfulness with, 90
    wariness of, 10
    women's choice of, 102
driving
    confusion while, 8
    dependency on others for, 58
    difficulties/fears, 13, 20, 26, 66, 94, 110
    loss of ability, 10, 67
    minimization of, 8
    seizure during, 23
dysthymia, 63

education, about epilepsy
    of family/friends, 86, 103
    teachers' need for, 87
EEG testing, 25, 82–83
embarrassment
    of family, 47–48
    freedom from, 73
    with friends, 48, 86
    at memory loss, 87, 109
    of public seizure, 13, 27, 64, 71

Index

emotional issues
  abuse, 9
  creating distance, 12
  feelings of guilt, 79
  influence of HRT, 109
  lack of maturity, 72
  lack of regard for others, 54
  lack of sustenance, 77
  security/confidence, 17
  terror/confusion, 54
  trauma from seizures, 56
emotional regard, lack of, 54
employers
  accommodation by, 52
  support by, 17, 95
employment
  difficulties maintaining, 38
  lack of difficulties with, 101–102
encouragement
  by doctors, 38
  by family, 22, 27–28
  by friends, 27–28
  by husband, 37, 81
epilepsy
  fear of word, 27
  positive side to, 11, 48–49, 97
  self-questioning about, 59
Epilepsy Foundation, 63

families
  acceptance by, 46, 80
  acceptance difficulties of, 11–12
  coping with children's seizures,
    13–14
  education of, 86
  encouragement by, 22
  history of epilepsy, 23
  increased sensitivity of, 85
  patience of, 21
  positive support from, 5–6, 16
  support from, 5–6, 85
fatigue
  from medication, 10, 46, 101
fears
  of admission of epilepsy, 2–3
  attempts at hiding, 61

doctors assuagement of, 102
  of driving, 66
  for experience of families/friends, 11,
    80, 86
  of having children, 3, 22–23,
    32, 34
  of marital difficulties, 3
  of medication, 40
  of parents, 24–25
  of rejection, 68
  reluctance for sharing, 3
  at schools, of students, 59
  of seizures, 26, 34, 55, 65, 99
  of sexuality issues, 50
  of word epilepsy, 27
first seizures, 9, 13, 19, 21, 24–25, 38–39,
    61, 67, 97, 114, 115–116
friends
  education of epilepsy for, 86, 103
  influence of epilepsy on, 74
  loss of, 48, 83, 88, 95
  patience of, 21, 106
  seizures witnessed by, 79
  steadfastness of, 83
  supportiveness of, 83, 86, 97

God
  desire for closeness to, 62
  prayer for no seizure to, 78, 89
  praying to for answers, 100
  presence of, 55
  thankfulness to, 26, 41, 65, 94
grand mal (tonic-clonic) seizures, 5,
    17–18, 35, 39, 42, 57, 61, 66, 78, 94,
    96, 100, 114–115
gratefulness
  for freedom from seizures, 36
  for spouse, 16
  for support group, 4
  for support of family/friends, 10, 16
  for trustworthy doctors, 16, 23
guilt
  of financial burden, 99
  at leaving early, 20–21
  for low sexual desire, 113
  self-imposed, 61, 79

Index

129

happiness
  at being alive, 30, 38
  at special school, 14
  of spouse, at seizure decrease, 106
heat sensitivity, 84
hirsutism, as medication side effect, 30–31
honesty
  about seizures, 17, 34, 37
  of doctor, 86, 116–117
hormone issues. *See also* menopause/
    perimenopause
  changes/imbalances of, 16, 31–32, 56,
    103–106, 109
  hormone replacement therapy (HRT),
    29, 105–106
  hormone-sensitive seizures, 117
husbands
  concerns about having children, 21, 32
  difficulty/pain of, 6
  hiding epilepsy from, 60, 65
  loving support from, 6–7
  as parental figure, 57
  patience of, 54–55
  protectiveness of, 8, 20
  resentment of, 57
  shame of, 60
  stability of relationship with, 83–84
  supportiveness of, 6–7, 17, 27, 33,
    65–66, 99, 102
  unmet expectations of, 35–36
  witnessing of seizures by, 19

independence
  fear of loss of, 9
  as foundational problem, 50
  as goal, 12
  growth of, 99
  loss of, 26–27, 32, 36, 51, 55, 67, 74,
    87, 95
  maintenance of, 29
  regaining of, 17
isolation, feelings of, 32, 62, 73, 116

marital issues. *See also* pregnancy issues
  difficulty/pain of spouses, 6
  falling apart of marriage, 36, 76

hiding illness, 3, 65–66
  keeping marriage strong, 8, 37, 54–55,
    65–66
  lesbian relationship, 9–12
  marriage *vs.* staying single,
    14–15
medical care disparity, male *vs.*
    female, 5
medication. *See also* side effects, of
    medication
  and appetite, 87, 114–115
  birth defect risks from, 78
  as cause of seizure, 15
  and cognitive functioning, 10, 58
  decisions for taking, 23–24
  effect on sexual desire, 10–11
  effect on unborn child, 16
  fatigue as side effect, 10, 46, 101
  improvements in, 77
  successfulness of, 6
  and work output, 12
meditation, 107
memory loss, 39, 52–53, 71, 87, 100,
    106–107
menopause/perimenopause, 26, 56.
    See also hormone issues
  and increased seizures, 17, 29, 40
  and seizures, 104–105, 106
menstruation issues
  irregularities of, 20, 113, 120
  side effects of medication, 110
mood swings, 6, 8, 75, 83
myoclonic seizures, 115

near-death experiences, 54
nervousness/stress-induced seizures, 9
normal
  attempt at appearing, 3, 41
  desire for being/feeling, 17, 89,
    102
  dreamlike staring as, 35
  family *vs.* person with epilepsy's
    perception of, 12
  return of senses to, 45
nutritional supplementation, 16, 20,
    25–26

Index

parents
  acceptance by children, 7, 59
  concerns of, 18–19, 26, 101, 111
  conference attendance by, 12
  confidence of, 21
  dealing with child's epilepsy, 20
  difficulties of, 11
  fears of, 24–25
  shame of, 20, 46, 76
patience
  of family/friends, 21, 100
  of husband, 54–55, 100
  with self, 98
petit mal seizures, 45, 61–62, 114
physical abuse, 9
positive side, to epilepsy
  increasing openness/sensitivity to
    others, 48–49
  support of family/friends/partners,
    11, 97
post-traumatic stress syndrome, 101
pregnancy issues
  birth defect fears, 3, 22–23
  decision against children, 13, 15
  doctors, for vs against, 7
  influence of medication, 16
  success having healthy children, 17
protection
  by Americans With Disabilities Act,
    27, 50, 104
  by spouses, 8, 20

questions
  of friends, about epilepsy, 13, 33–34,
    49
  of self, about epilepsy, 58, 83, 118–119
  of women, about HRT, 105, 106

rest
  importance of, 79
  and need for naps, 75
  paramedics suggestion for, 25
risks
  of birth defects, 78, 86
  of pregnancy, 15, 22–23
  of seizures, 57

school experiences
  avoidance of going, 72
  concerns of supervisors, 56
  fears of others, 59
  going back to school, 81–82
  seizures at, 21, 23, 55, 88, 114
  taunting by students, 30–31
seizures. See also first seizures; grand mal
    (tonic-clonic) seizures; myoclonic
    seizures
  abuse-induced, 9
  as cause of depression, 75, 79
  dreamlike feelings during, 34
  evening-into-nighttime, 6
  hormone-sensitive seizures, 117
  influence on senses, 45
  medication allergy induced, 15
  nervousness/stress-induced, 9
  return of after absence, 26–28
  at school, 21, 23, 55, 88, 114
  self-injury during, 41
  sleep only, 14, 104
  stress-induction of, 9, 105
  unpredictability of, 26, 41
  witnessing by others, 19, 55
self-acceptance, 15, 17, 38, 60, 63,
    85–86, 98, 103
self-confidence, 50, 67–68, 73, 99, 100
self-pitying, 28, 79, 89
senses, influence of seizures on, 45
sensitivity
  of family, 85
  to heat, 84
  towards others, 48, 110
sexual issues
  abuse, 9, 50
  avoidance of sexual interaction, 63
  effect of medication, 10–11, 71
  excessive demands by husband, 35
  fears about, 50
  lack of understanding about, 49–50, 74
  loss of desire, 10, 69, 76–77,
    100, 113
shame
  disavowing of, 93
  husband's causing of, 60

Index

131

shame (*continued*)
  of parents, 20, 46, 76
  by self, 32, 58, 61, 102–103
  of spouse, 60
siblings
  with epilepsy, 23
  support from, 28, 81
side effects, of medication
  balance difficulties, 47
  cognitive loss, 58
  decreased work output, 12, 77
  depression, 103
  fatigue, 101
  loss of sex drive, 10
  memory loss, 39
  menstrual irregularities, 110
  mood swings, 75
sleep deprivation EEG testing, 25
sleep-only seizures, 14, 104
slowing down, 33, 58, 110
smells
  of ammonia, 9
  of burning rubber/skunks, 109
stress
  and feelings of failure, 11
  from having seizures, 23
  and induction of seizures, 9, 105
  reduction strategies, 16, 27–28,
    33, 86–87
  spousal sharing of, 57
suicide, of husband, 80–81
support
  asking for, 11
  from coworkers, 67, 86, 110
  from doctors, 16, 41
  from employers, 17, 95
  of parent with epilepsy, by children, 17
  from family, 5–6, 16, 85
  from friends, 86
  from husbands, 6–7, 17, 27, 33, 65–66,
    99, 102
  lack of, 67, 77, 86

  from parents, 28
  from partners, 10
  from self, 6, 52
  from siblings, 28, 81
  spousal difficulties with, 6
  from spouses, 6–7, 16
  womens' groups, 4
support groups, 4
surgery
  for brain tumor removal, 56
  choice for having, 102
  recommendation by doctor, 38
  for seizure control, 35–36

teachers
  attitudes towards epilepsy, 21,
    112–113
  need for epilepsy education of, 87
  working as, 27, 55
temporal lobe epilepsy, 9
therapy
  for regaining of self-confidence, 12, 61
  seeking truth from, 63
tonic-clonic seizures. *See* grand mal
    (tonic-clonic) seizures
trance experience, 23
treatments
  delays due to lack of insurance, 11
  family discussions about, 50
  improvements in, 77
  lack of knowledge about, 48
  living with lack of, 72
  wariness of, 10
truth
  from doctors, about medication, 91
  seeking of, through therapy, 63

vitamin supplementation, 16, 20, 25–26

wariness, of doctors, 10
Women and Epilepsy program, 117
workplace accommodations, 52

Index